Thyroid Diet Plan

Charles Thompson

Copyright© 2021by Charles Thompson

 The information herein is offered for informational purposes solely, and is universal as so. The presentation of the information is without contract or any type of guarantee assurance. The trademarks that are used are without any consent, and the publication of the trademark is without permission or backing by the trademark owner. All trademarks and brands within this book are for clarifying purposes only and are the owned by the owners themselves, not affiliated with this document.

Index

Thyroid Diet Plan

Introduction

We often hear about the thyroid gland without necessarily knowing its exact function, so much so that in many cases, we ignore this gland until something starts to malfunction. The thyroid gland is as small as it is powerful, is characterized by a butterfly shape, and is located on the front of the neck. About 50 million US citizens have thyroid problems. Many people are unaware that fatigue, overweight, rapid heartbeat, and more could be due to this tiny gland's malfunction. One or more of these disorders should contact your doctor: he will recommend the proper tests (often a simple blood sample is enough) to understand if the cause is, for example, hypothyroidism or hyperthyroidism. In this case, nutrition can be an excellent ally to keep the thyroid under control and live with it in the best possible way. An articulated plan, a very specific menu (as well as the use of supplements and techniques for stress management) for this gland that works poorly, too much, or is inflamed. The goal is to favor the rebalancing of altered biomechanisms and physiological ones, bringing to the table the micronutrients essential for the optimal synthesis of thyroid hormones. Well to know, the diet must be customized according to each of us's physical and psychological characteristics; therefore, this guide wants to give you useful tips and recipes that help control the thyroid in a general way. The consultation with your doctor and then with the nutritionist must be the first steps to take to keep your thyroid under control.

Chapter 1: What is thyroid?

The thyroid is an endocrine gland located in the front of the neck, in front of the trachea, which gives it a characteristic "butterfly" appearance (the wings correspond to the right and left lobes). Despite its small size, the thyroid performs fundamental functions for our health: thyroid hormones control metabolic activities and are responsible for most of the body's cells' proper functioning. The thyroid regulates neuropsychic development, body growth, metabolism, cardiovascular function, bone formation, and growth from the first weeks of life. Not only that: it is always this gland that influences mood, muscle strength, fertility, and more. The thyroid tissue is organized into many thyroid follicles, the walls of which consist of a single layer of follicular cells (thyrocytes). Inside the follicles, there is a very viscous substance, the colloid, in which the synthesized hormones are accumulated and released from it, according to the needs of the organism. Finally, interleaved between the follicles are the parafollicular cells, responsible for calcitonin production, a hormone responsible for maintaining the balance of calcium in the body.

How Does the Thyroid Gland Work?

Thyroid cells first produce a protein that acts as a precursor to thyroid hormones, called thyroglobulin. Thyroglobulin is particularly rich in an amino acid called tyrosine. This amino acid is essential because thyrocytes selectively take iodine from the blood and transport it to the follicular cavity. It binds to the tyrosine of thyroglobulin to give rise to the thyroid hormones T3 and T4.

Iodine is an essential trace element for thyroid function, as it is contained in both thyroid hormones; these hormones influence many organs and tissues' activity and have a broad spectrum of action on the metabolism of carbohydrates, fats, and proteins and also on growth processes.

In addition to iodine, it is important to remember that selenium also plays a crucial role in thyroid functioning. It is no coincidence that this trace element in the gland is higher than in any other organ in the body. Selenium protects thyroid cells from oxidative damage and, at the level of target organs, participates in the reactions that activate thyroid hormones.

Returning to the thyroid follicles' characteristics, it is essential to note that the colloid is present inside them, which is a thick liquid with a high protein concentration. The colloid represents a sort of "warehouse," in which the thyroid hormones are stored and from where they are released according to the organism's needs. For example, with exposure to cold, the thyroid releases its hormones, increasing the basal metabolic rate, thus raising oxygen consumption at the cellular level and body temperature.

Thyroid hormones: T4 and T3

The hormones T4 (tetraiodothyronine or thyroxine) and T3 (triiodothyronine) regulate the body's metabolism and are necessary for the organism's growth and normal development. T3 and T4 are produced by thyroid follicular cells in response to the modulation of TSH (thyroid-stimulating hormone).

Synthesis of Thyroid Hormones

Some elements are essential for the synthesis of thyroid hormones:

Iodine;

Tyrosine;

Thyroperoxidase (TPO).

Iodine

Iodine is essential for the thyroid's proper functioning, as it is present in the chemical structure of both thyroid hormones and plays a decisive role in controlling their production and release into the bloodstream. For this reason, it is very important to ensure a sufficient intake of the element, which occurs above all with the diet, that is through the consumption of certain foods, such as, for example, sea fish, crustaceans, or products containing iodized salt. An insufficient intake of iodine leads to impaired synthesis and reduced thyroid hormones concentrations, which can cause various clinical manifestations. The best known consequence of iodine deficiency is goiter, which is the enlargement of the thyroid gland.

As for the synthesis of thyroid hormones, the iodine taken from food is absorbed in the intestine, is extracted from the plasma, and concentrated in the follicular cells in the form of iodide (I-), with an active transport mechanism: the Na + simport / I- (NIS co-transports 2 sodium ions and 1 iodine against the electrochemical gradient). The iodide captured by the thyroid is stored inside the colloid, organized at I2 thanks to the enzyme thyroperoxidase (TPO).

Tyrosine

In the colloid, enzymes for the synthesis of T3 and T4 and thyroglobulin (Tg), which acts as a precursor for thyroid hormones, are also found. Thyroxine and triiodothyronine derive, in fact, from the amino acid tyrosine, and thyroglobulin (Tg) provides precisely the tyrosine residues necessary to form the skeleton of their chemical structure. All components for the synthesis of thyroid hormones are therefore stored in the colloid.

Thyroperoxidase

The phases of synthesis begin with the intervention of the enzyme thyroperoxidase (TPO), which catalyzes the iodination reaction of tyrosine: the addition of an iodide ion forms monoiodothyrosine (MIT), and the addition of a second iodide to the same molecule constitutes diiodotyrosine (DIT). MIT and DIT are nothing more than precursors of thyroid hormones: T4 derives from the condensation reaction between two molecules of DIT, while T3 is obtained from the condensation of one molecule of MIT and one of DIT.

The thyroid hormones thus formed are bound to thyroglobulin supports and are stored in the colloid before their release, for months after their formation. Curiously, the thyroid is the only endocrine gland that can accumulate hormones in the extracellular area before their release. When TSH binding stimulates endocytosis of the thyroglobulin-thyroid hormone complex in follicular cells, thyroglobulin support is enzymatically degraded, while thyroid hormones are released into the cells into the bloodstream.

What is the thyroid gland for?

The thyroid is an organ that controls many key functions of our body through thyroxine (T4), triiodothyronine (T3), and calcitonin. First of all, the thyroid regulates the metabolism, which is the complex of reactions that allows the organs to obtain the energy necessary to perform their functions correctly. In other words, the hormones produces a signal to the body how fast it needs to work and how it needs to use food and chemicals to make energy. Not only that: the thyroid intervenes in the growth and development processes of many tissues and stimulates cellular activities, optimizing, in particular, the functions of the cardiovascular system and the nervous system. Understanding how thyroid activity can affect most of the body's cells leads to understanding why thyroid hormones must be produced in adequate quantities.

What is the Role of Thyroid Hormones

The actions of T4 and T3 are extensive and range from the development of the central nervous system to body growth to the control of numerous metabolic functions.

1. Thermogenetic action

Thyroid hormones contribute fundamentally to the energy expenditure and the endogenous production of heat, directly regulating the basal metabolism. This consists of the body's energy expenditure in rest conditions and includes the minimum amount of energy necessary to maintain essential vital functions, such as breathing, blood circulation, and nervous system activities. If thyroid hormones increase, it accelerates metabolic activity in most tissues. The direct consequence is the increase in oxygen consumption and the speed of use of energy substances, with heat production, a phenomenon known as the thermogenic effect. Part of this effect is the direct action of the hormones T3 and T4 on the mitochondria, the cell's energy plants. Thyroid hormones stimulate the activity of some enzymes involved in oxidative phosphorylation reactions at the mitochondrial respiratory chain level, producing ATP and releasing energy in the form of heat. T3 and T4 increase most of the body's tissues (exceptions to be noted are brain, spleen, and gonads).

2. Effects on carbohydrate, lipid and protein metabolism

T3 and T4 intervene in the use of energy and the mobilization of energy reserves, intervening in the synthesis and degradation of carbohydrates, lipids, and proteins. As for glucose metabolism, these favor the intestinal absorption of sugars, enhancing insulin action. At concentrations lower than usual, thyroid hormones stimulate gluconeogenesis in the liver and muscles. This process converts glucose into glycogen or, otherwise, if present in higher concentrations, they promote glycogenolysis, with a hyperglycemic effect. In lipid metabolism, thyroid hormones are involved with different results depending on their dosage. In the case of thyroid hyperactivity, an increase in lipolysis may occur, with the depletion of the lipid deposit and an increase in the availability of fatty acids; conversely, a lack of thyroid hormones causes the opposite effect, that is lipogenesis, with the synthesis of adipose tissue, which, among other things, leads to an increase in body weight. Finally, thyroid hormones stimulate protein synthesis; however, if present in excess, they can cause the opposite effect, in the sense that they block protein synthesis and increase catabolism, i.e., proteins are converted into amino acids, often at the expense of muscle mass.

3. Effects on the cardiovascular system

- Thyroid hormones have significant effects on the cardiovascular system:

- They favor contractility and contribute to myocardial excitability;

- They increase the heart rate;

Vascular resistance decreases, dilating peripheral arterioles and contributing to venous return. All this has the purpose of guaranteeing the necessary oxygen supply to the tissues. To achieve this, thyroid hormones can also determine an increase in pulmonary ventilation, which, to be efficient, requires an increase in cardiac output, i.e., the heart is induced to pump more. These effects also follows the increase in renal function.

4. Effects on the central nervous system

Thyroid hormones are necessary for the development of the central nervous system in the fetus and in the first weeks of life because they play a very important role in the differentiation and growth of nerve structures, as well as ensuring normal brain development. A deficiency of T3 and T4 in childhood can lead to a form of irreversible brain damage called cretinism, characterized by incomplete development of the central nervous system and mental retardation. Thyroid hormones ensure correct synaptogenesis (growth of dendrites and axons) and myelination of nervous structures.

5. Effects on the reproductive system

Normal thyroid function is also essential for the reproductive system. Thyroid hormones influence the development and maturation of the testicles and ovaries, ensuring correct spermatogenesis and reproductive activity for men and the regularity of the menstrual cycle and pregnancy maintenance in women. Therefore, dysfunction of the thyroid gland can cause consequences, such as infertility, sexual problems, and menstrual disorders.

6. Other effects

Thyroid hormones:

-They increase intestinal motility;

-They favor the absorption of vitamin B12 and iron;

-They increase the synthesis of erythropoietin;

-They increase renal flow and glomerular filtration;

-They regulate the tropism of the skin and appendages;

-They stimulate the endogenous production of other hormones, including growth hormone or GH.

We can affirm that the thyroid hormones, rather than intervening in a single site of action, modulate multiple and coordinated activities, allowing to maintain the whole organism's normal physiological functions. Other specific biological effects vary from one tissue to another. It is worth adding that thyroid hormones are essential for growth hormone or GH action and produce sensitive effects on the musculoskeletal system, promoting bone remodeling and increasing muscle contraction capacity. Finally, many of the stimulating effects on metabolism are amplified by catecholamines, such as adrenaline and noradrenaline, which act synergistically with thyroid hormones.

Diseases of the Thyroid

Sometimes, the thyroid can increase or decrease its activity, producing hormones in excess or defect compared to the body's real needs, as in the case of hyperthyroidism and hypothyroidism. In addition to dysfunctions, the thyroid can be affected by morphological changes, as in the case of goiters and nodules, or it can be the site of inflammation and tumors.

Hyperthyroidism

Hyperthyroidism is a disorder associated with hyperfunction of the thyroid gland, that is, excessive production of thyroid hormones; since thyroid hormones are responsible for controlling metabolism, hyperthyroidism causes an increase in many metabolic activities in peripheral tissues. The most frequent symptoms are, in fact, weight loss, tachycardia, nervousness, tremors, insomnia, muscle weakness, increased sweating, and intolerance to heat. Sometimes, the patient has apparent signs, such as an enlarged thyroid gland and the eyeballs' bulging. The causes of thyroid overactivity are manifold. Hyperthyroidism can be, for example, the consequence of a hyperfunctioning thyroid nodule or Graves' disease, which consists of an autoimmune disease characterized by the production of autoantibodies that act like the TSH hormone, i.e.,, stimulating the thyroid.

Hypothyroidism

We talk, however, of hypothyroidism when the thyroid does not produce a number of thyroid hormones adequate to the needs of the organism. This may be due to both thyroid insufficiency and to an alteration of the balance between the thyroid, hypothalamus, and pituitary, as, for example, in the case of inappropriate TSH secretion. This determines, in addition to the reduction of metabolic processes, symptoms such as fatigue, slowing of reflexes, reduced appetite, and weight gain. The causes of hypothyroidism are diverse: iodine deficiency, autoimmune thyroid disease, outcomes of surgery, and neck irradiation.

Goiter

Another condition is goiter, which generally defines any increase in thyroid volume. The goiter can be uninodular or multinodular, if it affects, respectively, one or more areas, or it can be characterized by widespread enlargement of the whole gland. The enlargement of the thyroid gland can occur both in hyperthyroidism and hypothyroidism; bearing in mind that there are also goiters that do not modify thyroid function. In any case, the result is the appearance of a lump on the neck, which can even compress other nearby organs, making it difficult to swallow or breathe.

Thyroid nodules

The thyroid gland can also be affected by the formation of thyroid nodules. Their development is usually a phenomenon of a benign nature. Often, these small lumps localized on the thyroid do not alter its functionality and do not cause any symptoms but require a specific diagnostic evaluation to exclude both tumor pathologies and possible future dysfunctions.

Tumors of the thyroid gland

Both benign and malignant tumors can arise in the thyroid. Thyroid tumors, with rare exceptions, often have a benign clinical course. Therefore they can be controlled by therapy with excellent results.

Chapter 2: Thyroiditis

Thyroiditis is an inflammation of the thyroid gland and we can identify different forms of it, such as:

- acute (very rare and usually due to bacterial or parasitic infections)
- sub-acute (usually of viral origin),
- chronic (usually due to autoimmune, but not limited to):
- by Hashimoto,
- sporadic,
- postpartum,
- Riedel fibrous,
- from drugs.

The acute and sub-acute forms generally allow a complete recovery of thyroid function. The gland can hurt and be swollen if the thyroiditis is caused by an infection or trauma, unlike in cases where the cause is an autoimmune disorder or drugs. Young and middle-aged women are the population most at risk. However, some forms affect both men and women of any age. In some cases, hypothyroidism can begin even years after the onset of the disease, even if the thyroiditis has been treated. It is not possible to draw up a single list of typical symptoms of thyroiditis, as they are strictly dependent on the developed form and its phase; from a general point of view:

if thyroiditis causes slow and progressive destruction of thyroid cells (as in the case of Hashimoto), it results in a decrease in the levels of thyroid hormones in the blood; in this case, patients present with the symptoms of hypothyroidism:

- fatigue,
- weight gain,
- constipation,
- dry skin,
- depression
- and poor exercise tolerance.

If thyroiditis causes rapid and violent damage, the thyroid hormone stored in the gland is released suddenly, increasing the thyroid hormone levels in the blood. These patients will experience the symptoms of thyrotoxicosis, which are similar to hyperthyroidism:

- anxiety,
- insomnia,
- palpitations (rapid heartbeat),
- fatigue,
- weight loss
- and irritability.

Causes

The cause of thyroid inflammation is usually found in some form of attack on the gland, which causes inflammation and cell damage; the agent changes depending on the case and can be:

- antibodies produced by your body (in case of immune system disorders),
- microorganisms (viruses, bacteria, and parasites),
- diseases that cause fever,
- some medications

The most common case is the autoimmune form. Abnormal production of antibodies occurs, proteins that should typically protect us from external microorganisms. Instead, in some cases and for unknown reasons, mistake the thyroid for a target to attack. In some cases, the cause of thyroiditis remains unknown.

Risk factors

- Most thyroiditis forms are three to five times more prevalent in women than in men, possibly due to hormonal factors.
- With increasing age, the risk of developing the disease increases; the average age at the onset of the disease is usually between 30 and 50 years.
- This disease tends to be geographically connoted and seasonal. It tends to strike, especially in summer and autumn.
- A significant association has been shown between Hashimoto's thyroiditis and genetic causes.
- A variable percentage from 8% to 10% of pregnant women develops autoimmune thyroiditis, which has the same characteristics as Hashimoto's thyroiditis, but it will resolve completely after delivery.
- Pregnant women who test positive for thyroid antibodies in the first trimester have a 30-50% risk of developing thyroiditis after delivery.
- The intake of iodine seems to increase the risk of developing the problem in predisposed subjects, for causes still unknown.
- Radiation (for example, there was an increase in cases following Chernobyl).
- Infections.

Symptoms

Possible symptoms are numerous and often not very specific, so the disorder can be difficult to diagnose. Multiple variables affect the type and extent of symptoms, so this section is to be interpreted as a general description. The acute form is often characterized by a swelling of the neck, with the skin that is hot and red. There may be fever and swollen lymph nodes and only rarely other symptoms.

When the thyroid is inflamed, it often releases an excess of thyroid hormone, causing hyperthyroidism. Then, when there is no more thyroid hormone to dismiss, the body no longer has enough of it, and therefore we have hypothyroidism and may appear:

- fatigue,
- weight gain,
- confusion,
- depression,
- dry skin,
- constipation.

Other rarer symptoms include:

- swelling of the legs,
- widespread pain,
- decreased ability to concentrate.

In the event of more advanced cell damage, the following

can finally occur:

- swelling around the eyes,
- bradycardia (slow heart rate),
- drop in body temperature,
- heart failure.

On the other hand, if the damage to thyroid cells is acute, the thyroid hormone within the gland reaches the bloodstream causing symptoms of thyrotoxicosis, very similar to those of an overactive thyroid (hyperthyroidism):

- weight loss,
- irritability,
- anxiety,
- insomnia,
- tachycardia,
- constant sense of fatigue.

In the case of Hashimoto's thyroiditis, the appearance of goiter (an increase in the volume of the thyroid, often visible externally) is frequent, a phenomenon that occurs gradually.

In some cases, thyroiditis, particularly postpartum, can be completely asymptomatic.

Chapter 3: Diets and nutrition

Diet for HYPOTHYROIDISM

The ideal hypothyroidism diet consists of foods that help maintain proper thyroid function, therefore rich in iodine, selenium, and zinc. On the contrary, all processed and processed foods and soy-based foods should be avoided in the hypothyroidism diet because they compromise regular thyroid function. In particular, soy-based supplements reduce the effectiveness of hormone therapy prescribed by the doctor and should therefore be preferably avoided. Hypothyroidism slows down the metabolism, which is why it often coincides with weight gain. In the diet for hypothyroidism, we choose foods that help produce the hormones that the thyroid can no longer make.

Below is a table of recommended foods to limit or to avoid to better manage your diet for hypothyroidism:

Recommended foods	Foods to limit	Foods to avoid
Choose to introduce foods rich in selenium, an antioxidant nutrient useful for the production of hormones (the thyroid itself is made up of a part of selenium).	In moderate quantities, prefer foods rich in IODIUM that stimulate the thyroid gland (if consumed in excess they can worsen hypothyroidism or lead to	Avoid all SOY based foods including: soy milk, soy sauce, soy beans, tofu, seitan, miso. The isoflavones contained in

Foods rich in SELENIUM are for example: tuna, shrimp, beef, turkey, chicken, ham, eggs, oat flakes, wholemeal flour bread.	hyperthyroidism): cheeses, milk, ice cream, iodized table salt, saltwater fish (especially crustaceans, algae and molluscs), whole eggs.	soy, such as genistein and daidzein, cause a decrease in the production of hormones.
To be preferably included in the diet for hypothyroidism are also foods rich in ZINC such as: oysters, beef, crabs, cereals, pork, chicken, legumes, pumpkin seeds, yogurt.	These, on the other hand, are foods to be limited or avoided altogether. They are to be consumed necessarily cooked, as in the cooking process they lose anti-thyroid substances. These are cabbage, Brussels sprouts, Russian cabbage, broccoli and cauliflower.	Also avoid all processed and processed foods that only help to gain weight and do not offer necessary nutrients, among these we have: hot dogs, fast food in general.

Diet for HYPERTIROIDISM

Some of the people who develop Hashimoto's Thyroiditis experience an overactive thyroid condition (hyperthyroidism). So all the foods and advice just given regarding hypothyroidism are to be forgotten. The diet for hyperthyroidism is, in fact, a diet symmetrically opposite to that for hypothyroidism. Now the main problem is that the thyroid produces too many hormones, so you need to include foods that inhibit your diet's thyroid function.

Here is the summary table of the recommended foods to limit and avoid in the case of a Diet for Hyperthyroidism aimed at decreasing the production of hormones:

Recommended foods	Foods to limit	Foods to avoid
Fresh fruit is recommended, especially pear, peach, papaya and mango.	Sea fish maximum 2 times a week.	Eliminate foods rich in IODIUM that stimulate the thyroid: cheeses, milk, ice cream, iodized table salt, saltwater fish (especially shellfish, swordfish, seaweed and molluscs), whole eggs.

Include millet, pine nuts, flax seeds and peanuts in your diet for hyperthyroidism	ZINC-rich foods such as beef, fortified cereals, pork, chicken, yogurt, can also be moderately included in the diet for hyperthyroidism.	Avoid coffee, tea, some spices like cinnamon
The consumption of legumes in general such as soy, chickpeas, beans, lentils is recommended.	Use salt in moderation.	Avoid the consumption of tasty or too salty products such as: chips, salty snacks of all kinds, spicy sauces, smoked cheeses, fatty meats.
We recommend these vegetables in generous quantities: broccoli, rocket, cabbage, Brussels sprouts, cauliflower, radishes, peppers, carrots.	Carbohydrates should not be excessively present in the hyperthyroid diet, possibly they should be whole carbohydrates.	Also avoid sushi, as it is rich in carbohydrates and saltwater fish.

Herbal teas of valerian and lemon balm in the afternoon and / or after dinner, recommended to promote sleep and relaxation compromised by excessive hormone production.		To avoid pistachios, almonds, garlic, cashews.

Exercise and avoid alcohol and smoking

A healthy lifestyle helps you stay fit and healthy, and your thyroid benefits too. Although scientific studies do not give specific information on the effects of physical activity and alcohol on thyroid function, it is still good to stay active even with a simple 20-30 minute walk a day and limit alcohol consumption. Some data in the literature would suggest a possible link between thyroid function and cigarette smoking. In particular, the negative effect of smoking on ocular complications of autoimmune hyperthyroidism is known.

Chapter 4: Recipes for hypothyroidism

Breakfast

•Pistachio cookies

Ingredients:
- 350 g of Manitoba flour
- 100 g of chopped pistachios
- 150 g of corn malt
- 75 ml of corn oil
- 150 ml of soya milk
- 12 g of cream of tartar yeast
- a pinch of cinnamon
- a pinch of salt

Put the dry ingredients in a container: flour, pistachios, baking powder, cinnamon, salt, and stir. In a mug, mix the malt, oil and 100 ml of soy milk. Pour them over the dry ingredients, work with one hand in a circular direction, mixing the dough and slowly incorporate the rest of the soy milk until the mixture is solid, soft and a little sticky. Let it rest for 15 minutes. Take small amounts of the dough and form balls the size of a walnut. Arrange them on the baking tray and bake them in a preheated oven at 190 ° C for 18-20 minutes or until golden.

• Muffins with bananas and carrots

Ingredients:
- 200 g of wholemeal flour
- 1 banana
- 1 medium carrot
- milk
- 60 g of honey
- 50 g of vegetable butter
- 1 egg
- 2 teaspoons of lemon juice
- 2 teaspoons of cream of tartar
- 1 pinch of salt

Gather the chopped butter, honey, and five tablespoons of milk in a small saucepan. Heat them over low heat, stirring until they are homogeneous. Let them cool down a bit. Meanwhile, mash the banana with a fork and coarsely grate the carrot. Mix them in a bowl with the flour, cream of tartar, and salt; gradually incorporate the previously prepared mixture and lemon juice. Finally, add the beaten egg. If necessary, dilute with a bit of milk to have a soft dough. Pour it into paper cups and bake at 180 degrees for about 20 minutes. Allow the muffins to cool on a wire rack before enjoying them.

•

Light pancake

Ingredients:
- **100 g of egg whites**
- **125 g of Greek yogurt**
- **80 g of wholemeal flour**
- **2 tablespoons of honey**
- **2 tablespoons of skim milk**
- **1 tablespoon of seed oil**
- **1 teaspoon of baking powder for cakes**
- **1/4 teaspoon of baking soda**
- **1/2 vanilla bean**

TO SERVE
- **honey**
- **blueberries or other fruit to taste**

To make the light pancakes, first, collect the egg whites in a bowl. Beat them with a hand whisk for 30 seconds. Add the Greek yogurt, vanilla seeds, honey, and oil. Work everything until you get a homogeneous cream. Add the wholemeal flour, sifted with baking powder and baking soda, and mix it by slowly adding the milk. You will need to obtain a smooth and homogeneous batter with a slightly thick but not too thick consistency. Grease a non-stick pan with the seed oil and heat it well, removing the excess oil with kitchen paper. Pour a ladle of batter and let it spread out into a disc. When you notice large bubbles appear on the surface, turn the pancake and continue cooking on the other side. When cooked, transfer to a plate. Proceed in this way until the batter is used up. Serve the light pancakes warm with honey and blueberries.

•Dark chocolate, almond and matcha mini-cupcake without baking

Ingredients:
- **200 g of 70% dark chocolate**
- **1 large handful of shelled almonds**
- **matcha tea**
- **a few pinches of Himalayan salt**
- **a few pinches of vanilla powder**

Melt the dark chocolate in a double boiler. As soon as it has liquefied, add the chopped or chopped almonds, 2 teaspoons of matcha tea, salt, vanilla, and mix well. Pour the mixture into small molds for chocolates or into molds for molds in which you have inserted cupcake cases. Let it cool to room temperature or in the refrigerator. When the cakes have completely solidified, decorate them with a sprinkling of matcha tea.

•Lemon cookies

Ingredients:
•2 cups of wholemeal flour
•2 cups of white flour
•3/4 cup corn oil
•a pinch of salt
•the grated peel of 3 organic lemons

For the dough's excellent result and speed up the times, it is good to use cold, iced water and work the dough as little as possible. Gather the flours, salt, and peel of 3 lemons in a bowl, pour the oil in the center, and enough water to obtain a thick and creamy mixture. The dough should be rolled out immediately and roughly cut into diamond shapes to get many irregular biscuits. Bake in a hot oven at 200 degrees for 10 minutes.

•Dried fruit tarts

Ingredients:
- **130 g of wholemeal flour**
- **100 g of almond flour**
- **2 tablespoons of rice malt**
- **2 tablespoons of corn oil**
- **4 tablespoons of vegetable milk (almonds, oats, rice)**
- **half a teaspoon of vanilla powder**
- **1 teaspoon of cream of tartar**
- **1 pinch of salt**
- **200 g of mixed dried fruit (apricots, raisins, plums pitted)**
- **10 almonds cut in half lengthwise**
- **the peel of 1 orange**
- **2 star anise berries**

Wash the dried fruit and put it covered with water in a saucepan for a few hours. Add the anise, orange peel, and a pinch of salt. Cook gently until the fruit is tender and dry, removing the aniseed at the end of cooking. If necessary, transfer it to a colander so that it dries well. Prepare the dough by mixing the dry ingredients (flour, vanilla, cream of tartar, salt) in a bowl; add the malt, oil, and milk already mixed. Work everything just enough to obtain a homogeneous dough that you will roll out into a thin sheet. Line the molds with the dough and grease them with oil. Stuffed with fruit, decorate the surface with almonds and bake at 160 ° for about 20 minutes, until the dough is golden brown.

• Turmeric pumpkin bread

Ingredients
- **700 grams of wholemeal flour**
- **350 grams of pumpkin**
- **200 grams of sourdough**
- **half a cup of sunflower oil**
- **1 tablespoon of whole sea salt**
- **1 tablespoon of turmeric**
- **250-300 ml of warm water**

Steam the pumpkin and mash it with a potato masher, collecting the past in a bowl. Add the rest of the ingredients and work the dough vigorously on a pastry board for 15 minutes. Grease a pan with a diameter of 30 cm, arrange the dough by covering it with a cloth, and let it rise in the heat for 2 hours. Meanwhile, preheat the oven to 230 ° C, or 210 ° C if it is ventilated, placing a steel basin filled with water in the lower part. Brush the dough with water and bake the bread. After 30 minutes, lower the temperature by 30 ° C and continue cooking for another 15 minutes. Remove from the oven and allow to cool before enjoying.

•Pear, chocolate and hazelnut muffins

Ingredients:
•3 cups of kamut flour
•2 tablespoons of cream of tartar
•half a teaspoon of ground cinnamon
•half a cup of toasted hazelnuts
•half a cup of dark chocolate
•half a cup of sunflower oil
•half a cup of wheat malt
•1 and a half cups of soy milk
•1 large cup of pears cut into small pieces
•1 pinch of salt

Mix the flour, salt, cream of tartar, and cinnamon in a bowl; in another, emulsify the oil with the malt and milk, then pour it into the first, mixing everything without mixing too much. Add the coarsely chopped hazelnuts and chocolate, the peeled and chopped pears. Spread the mixture into muffin cups and bake at 180 degrees for about 30 minutes.

•Date and almond cake

Ingredients:
- 230 g of flour 0
- 40 g of corn malt
- 40 ml of corn oil
- 5 g of fresh brewer's yeast
- 1 small teaspoon of vanilla powder
- the grated peel of 1/2 lemon
- 60 ml of warm water

For the date cream
- 500 g of pitted dates
- 350 ml of water
- 1 pinch of salt

To decorate
mixture of malt and hot water in a ratio of 3 to 1
- 20 g of flaked almonds

Wash the dates and cook covered and over low heat with water and a pinch of salt until the cooking liquid is completely absorbed. Blend and let the cream cool. Proceed by preparing the cake dough: melt the brewer's yeast in warm water and leave it aside. In the meantime, take a large bowl to put the flour, a pinch of salt, vanilla, and lemon peel. Make a hole in the center and stir in the corn oil and then, little by little, the yeast and malt. Then work the dough by combining all the ingredients, always with more energy, and helping yourself with a bit of flour until you have a ball free of lumps.

Flour a work surface and transfer the dough into it: knead it for about 5 minutes, with continuous and circular movements, until it is elastic and smooth. Let it rest for 30 minutes. With a rolling pin, make a sheet by pressing the dough, starting from the center and proceeding outwards. When you have obtained a disk of about 30 cm, place it on a baking sheet lined with parchment paper, and with your thumbs, press the internal corners of the pastry.

Orange Plumcake

Ingredients:
- 2 eggs at room temperature
- 170 g of granulated sugar
- 160 ml of orange juice
- 80 ml of seed oil
- 210 g of flour 00
- 50 g of potato starch
- 16 g of baking powder for cakes
- 1 pinch of cinnamon
- 2 organic blood oranges

Start preparing the orange plum cake by whipping the eggs with sugar and cinnamon in the planetary mixer or a large bowl until you get a frothy mixture. Add the finely grated zest of 1 orange and mix. Then add the seed oil and the orange juice, filtered through a colander, taking care to incorporate them well. Continue with the sifted flour together with the starch and baking powder. Pour half of the mixture into a 25x11 cm loaf pan. Place 4 or 5 thinly sliced orange halves on top, cover with the remaining mixture, and spread other orange slices in half on the surface. Transfer to a preheated oven at 180 degrees for about 45 minutes. At the end of cooking, do the classic "toothpick test" to make sure that the cake is ready. Remove the orange plum cake from the oven and let it cool completely before turning it out of the mold and serving.

Appetizer, Snack, Side dishes

•Grilled red cabbage with vegetable yogurt, almonds and turmeric

Ingredients:
- 1 medium red cabbage
- 200 g of natural and sugar-free vegetable yogurt
- 1 clove of garlic
- 1 handful of shelled almonds
- 1 teaspoon of turmeric powder
- dried rosemary, to decorate
- sesame oil
- freshly ground black pepper
- whole sea salt

Wash the red cabbage well and dry it. Cut it lengthwise, making slices about 1 cm thick and trying to keep them compact. Arrange them on a baking sheet lined with parchment paper, salt them lightly and place them under the preheated grill. Let them brown slightly, being careful not to burn them. In the meantime, coarsely chop the almonds, otherwise chop or cut into slices. Blend the yogurt with the peeled and sliced clove of garlic and a tablespoon of sesame oil. Finally, distribute the cabbage in the individual serving plates, pouring a little of the yogurt sauce, a thread of sesame oil, and the turmeric powder on each slice. Decorate with rosemary and serve immediately.

•Breaded broccoli

Ingredients:

- **2 stalks of broccoli**
- **bread crumbs**
- **1 teaspoon of thyme**
- **1 large egg**
- **1 clove of garlic**
- **2 tablespoons of oil**
- **salt and chilli**

Turn on the oven at 180 degrees. Remove the outer layer of the broccoli and slice the excellent stems to obtain discs. Finely chop the garlic and mix it with the breadcrumbs. Add the paprika, chili, and thyme. Mix well. Beat the egg in a bowl and salt it lightly. Pass the coins first in the egg and then in the breadcrumbs, coating them evenly. Line a baking sheet with parchment paper and brush it with oil. Distribute the coins and bake for 10-15 minutes, turning them once. Remove the coins from the oven and serve them immediately.

•Spring onions, and roasted cumin peppers

Ingredients:
- **600 g of spring onions**
- **600 g of red peppers**
- **½ garlic**
- **½ teaspoon of crushed cumin**
- **1 tablespoon of apple cider vinegar**
- **2 tablespoons of lemon juice**
- **3 tablespoons of vinegar**
- **salt**
- **3 tablespoons of chopped parsley**

Clean the spring onions, keeping the green part; wash the peppers and leave them whole. Arrange everything on a baking sheet lined with baking paper together with the washed but unpeeled garlic. Bake at 180 degrees until all the vegetables are soft. Let them cool down. Open the peppers, remove seeds and ribs, cut them into slices. Thinly slice the spring onions. Puree the garlic and put it in a bowl. Add the lemon juice, vinegar, oil, salt, and cumin. Beat well with a fork. Arrange spring onions and peppers on a serving dish and toss with the prepared sauce. Sprinkle with parsley, let it rest for about ten minutes, and serve.

•Chickpea crepes with vegetables and vegan pesto mayonnaise

Ingredients:
Ingredients for crepes:
•200 g of chickpea flour
•300-350 g of cold water
•90 ml of extra virgin olive oil
•a pinch of salt
•a pinch of pepper

Ingredients for the vegetable filling:
•3 medium carrots
•a bunch of fresh chard leaves
•a clove of garlic
•a teaspoon of chopped fresh thyme
•extra virgin olive oil to taste
•a pinch of salt

Ingredients for the mayonnaise
•a jar of organic basil pesto
•200 ml of unsweetened soy milk
•300-350 ml of sunflower oil
•a pinch of salt
•a teaspoon of cream mustard
•the juice of half a lemon

We prepare the dough for the crepes by homogeneously mixing the chickpea flour, water, oil, salt, and pepper to obtain a fluid and lump-free batter. Let it sit for 20 minutes. Meanwhile, wash and peel the carrots, cutting them into thin strips of the size you want.

Wash and drain the chard leaves, coarsely chopping the larger leaves if necessary. Heat two tablespoons of oil in a non-stick pan with garlic and thyme, then add the vegetables and cook quickly for 10 minutes. Add salt and cover, leaving the filling warm. Now put all the ingredients for the mayonnaise in a blender, except the pesto. Blend until you get a thick and homogeneous cream. Taste and season with salt. Place the mayonnaise in a small bowl and mix with 2 tablespoons of basil pesto. At this point, you can proceed in the composition of your crepes: then heat a non-stick pan with a drizzle of extra virgin olive oil and place a little batter starting from the center. Cook both sides well and place in a tray. Repeat the operation until the batter is used up. Then take an open crepe on a plate and stuff it in the center with the vegetables and mayonnaise. Close by forming a cylinder. Repeat with all the crepes and serve in a serving dish.

• Sauteed spinach with dried fruit

Ingredients:
- **500 g of spinach**
- **50 g of dried apples**
- **50 g of raisins**
- **a little pine nuts**
- **1 clove of garlic**
- **extra virgin olive oil as needed**
- **Salt to taste.**

Soak the apples and raisins for about 20 minutes in warm water. Clean and wash the spinach. Blanch them in lightly salted water for a few minutes. Drain them by squeezing them well, and cut them coarsely. Fry the garlic in a pan greased with oil, add the spinach, and after a while, the raisins and well-squeezed apples, pine nuts, and salt. Let it cook over high heat for a few minutes, season with salt, and serve the spinach hot.

• Carrot puree with green olives

Ingredients:
- **500 g of spinach**
- **50 g of dried apples**
- **50 g of raisins**
- **a little pine nuts**
- **1 clove of garlic**
- **extra virgin olive oil as needed**
- **Salt to taste.**

Soak the apples and raisins for about 20 minutes in warm water. Clean and wash the spinach. Blanch them in lightly salted water for a few minutes. Drain them by squeezing them well, and cut them coarsely. Fry the garlic in a pan greased with oil, add the spinach, and after a while, the raisins and well-squeezed apples, pine nuts, and salt. Let it cook over high heat for a few minutes, season with salt, and serve the spinach hot.

•Turmeric chickpeas sauteed with radicchio, dates and almonds

Ingredients:
- 1 head of red radicchio
- •400 g of cooked chickpeas
- 1 clove of garlic
- 1 tablespoon of turmeric powder
- extra virgin olive oil
- ½ teaspoon of cumin powder
- 7-8 pitted dates
- 1 handful of shelled almonds
- sea salt

In a heavy-bottomed pan, heat a little oil and brown the peeled and chopped garlic. Add the chickpeas, let them flavor, and add turmeric and cumin, stir, and lightly salt. Cook over high heat for about a minute, stirring constantly. Add the peeled and cleaned radicchio; it must wither for a couple of minutes. Just before removing from the heat, add the dates cut into small pieces. Complete with the chopped almonds, a drizzle of extra virgin olive oil, and bring to the table.

•Fennel in orange cream

Ingredients:
- **2 medium fennel**
- **1 cup of cashews**
- **125 ml of orange juice**
- **2 teaspoons of dried mint**
- **1 pinch of chilli**
- **1 tablespoon of oil**
- **½ teaspoon of salt**
- **1 teaspoon of agave syrup**

Wash the fennel, cut them into four parts, and, using a mandolin, slice them finely. Sprinkle it with salt and let it rest. Meanwhile, prepare the cream. Put the cashews in the blender with the orange juice, mint, chili pepper, oil, salt, and agave syrup and mix until the mixture is fluid and without lumps. Drain the fennel water and season with the cream.

Red cabbage with spices

Ingredients:
- ½ red cabbage
- 3 apples
- 1 orange
- 3 tablespoons of raisins
- 3 tablespoons of pine nuts
- ½ glass of apple vinegar
- 2 tablespoons of oil
- 2 cloves
- cinnamon powder
- nutmeg
- salt

Cut the cabbage into thin strips and toss it in a heavy-bottomed pot with oil until it "sweats." Add the orange juice, the thinly sliced peel, and the apple vinegar. Lower the heat and add the apples cut into small pieces, the cloves, the previously soaked raisins, and a nice pinch of salt to the pot. Mix well, cover, and cook for about 40 minutes or until the cabbage is very soft. During the last 10 minutes of cooking, add the spices and pine nuts. It is even better to eat the next day.

• Brussels sprouts with chestnuts and currants

Ingredients:
- **350 g of Brussels sprouts**
- **12-15 boiled chestnuts**
- **2-3 sprigs of red currant**
- **1 clove of garlic**
- **oil**
- **salt**
- **pepper**
- **a few sprigs of thyme**
- **a few drops of balsamic vinegar**

Cook the sprouts in lightly salted boiling water for a few minutes, until tender; drain well and pour into a pan where the oil has been flavored with the crushed garlic. Brown briefly, then add the chestnuts and mix again. Season with pepper, thyme, and a few drops of balsamic vinegar. Garnish with the currants and serve immediately.

Soups and salad

- **Black lentil cream**

Ingredients:
- **200 g of black lentils**
- **1 onion**
- **1 clove of garlic**
- **1 carrot**
- **1 stick of celery**
- **10 cm of kombu seaweed**
- **bay leaf, rosemary, sage**
- **salt and pepper**
- **chili pepper**
- **2 tablespoons of oil**

To garnish
- **1 diced carrot**
- **chopped parsley**

Dice the celery and carrot, slice the onion and garlic. Heat a saucepan, pour in the oil, and immediately sauté the latter for a couple of minutes, stirring constantly. Add the remaining vegetables and a pinch of chili. Continue cooking for a few minutes, then add the washed lentils, a liter of water, the kombu, pepper, and a bunch prepared with bay leaves, rosemary, and sage. Cover and cook gently for 40 minutes. Remove the seaweed and the aromas. Add salt, blend, let it boil again for a couple of minutes, and turn off. Boil a little water, add a pinch of salt and blanch the carrot as a garnish for 3 minutes. Serve the soup decorating it with cubes and parsley. Complete with a drizzle of raw oil.

•Leek and pineapple salad

Ingredients:
• **2 medium leeks (white only)**
• **150 g of clean pineapple**
• **1 head of curly salad**
• **1 heart of celery**
• **1 lemon**
• **3 tablespoons of oil**
• **50 g of cashews**
• **1 sprig of fresh mint**
• **salt and chilli**

Wash the salad and dry it, then place it in a large bowl. Add the celery rinsed under the tap and sliced. Then add the leek, cleaned and cut into slices, the pineapple cut into cubes, chili pepper according to taste, the lemon juice, the oil, and salt. Stir well. Coarsely chop the cashews and distribute them on the salad together with the coarsely chopped mint.

•Pumpkin and beetroot salad

Ingredients:
•400 grams of pumpkin
•4 beets
•1 tablespoon of balsamic vinegar
•1 tablespoon of black sesame seeds
•2 bunches of rocket
•200 grams of cottage cheese
•extra virgin olive oil to taste
•Salt to taste.
•pepper as needed.

Put the whole beets with the peel in a baking dish with half a glass of water, cover, and bake in the oven at 180 ° for about an hour until they become soft (you may need more water). Also, bake the pumpkin cut into small pieces, with oil, salt, and pepper, until tender and golden. When the beets have cooled sufficiently, peel them and cut them into wedges. Mix salt, pepper, balsamic vinegar, and oil. Combine the beets, pumpkin, and rocket in a salad bowl. Add the sauce and sprinkle with sesame seeds and crumbled goat cheese or smoked tofu cut into small cubes.

•Potato and leek soup

Ingredients:
- **2 large potatoes**
- **2 large leeks**
- **800 ml of water**
- **1 shallot**
- **3-4 tablespoons of extra virgin olive oil**
- **1 teaspoon of powdered vegetable broth**
- **1 tablespoon of dried oregano**
- **a few pinches of whole sea salt**
- **a few pinches of freshly ground white pepper**

For the pumpkin seed pesto:
- **3-4 tablespoons of pumpkin seeds**
- **a handful of fresh parsley**
- **half a clove of garlic**
- **a few drops of lemon juice**
- **a tablespoon of extra virgin olive oil**
- **a pinch of whole sea salt**
- **a spoonful of water**

Heat the oil over high heat in a thick-bottomed pot and let the chopped shallot dry out. Add the diced potatoes, oregano, pepper, and add salt by cooking for a few minutes, constantly stirring to prevent the potatoes from sticking to the bottom. Pour the water and the broth powder into the pot, mix, cover, lower the heat and cook for another 15-20 minutes. Add the thinly sliced leek and continue to cook without a lid for about another 10 minutes, until tender.

You can cook even longer if you want a creamier texture.
In the meantime, prepare the pumpkin seed pesto by
finely chopping the seeds with the parsley and garlic and
mixing everything with the lemon juice, oil, salt, and
water, with the help of an immersion mixer. . When it is
time to serve the soup, distribute it in individual bowls
and complete with a drizzle of oil and a desired amount of
pesto.

•Cauliflower with olives and dried tomatoes
Ingredients:
- **800 g of cauliflower**
- **1 large red onion**
- **12 dried tomatoes**
- **16 pitted black olives**
- **oil**
- **salt**
- **pepper**

Rehydrate the dried tomatoes in warm water for 15
minutes, cut the onion into slices and the cauliflower into
florets. Drain the tomatoes and cut them into slices. Heat
a pan, add the oil and onion, sauté for a few minutes,
stirring constantly, then add the cauliflower, tomatoes,
and olives. Salt, pepper, pour a drop of water, cover, and
stew for 10-12 minutes. Remove any liquid and serve.

• Chestnut and chickpea soup

Ingredients:
- **200 g of dried chestnuts**
- **200 g of chickpeas**
- **2 tablespoons of chopped parsley**
- **1 teaspoon of dried thyme**
- **1 clove of garlic**
- **2 shallots**
- **4 tablespoons of dry white wine**
- **1 teaspoon of fennel seeds**
- **1 bay leaf**
- **1 chilli**
- **3 tablespoons of oil**
- **salt**

Soak chickpeas and chestnuts separately for one night. Drain and rinse them. Put the first courses in a pressure cooker with the bay leaf and garlic. Cover them with water and cook for 15 minutes from the whistle. As soon as possible, carefully open the pot, add the chestnuts, and then the fennel seeds and salt. Continue the pressure cooking for another 15 minutes. Meanwhile, peel and chop the shallots with the chili. Sauté them in a pan with the thyme and wine. As soon as they begin to smell, turn them off and add them to the contents of the pot, which you will always have uncovered with caution. Continue cooking for another 10 minutes. Remove the bay leaf and blend almost all the chickpeas and chestnuts, using hot water if needed. Season with salt and season with oil. Serve the soup hot.

• Spiced pumpkin cream

Ingredients:
- **1.5 kg of pumpkin**
- **1 shallot**
- **vegetable broth or water to taste**
- **1 teaspoon of curry powder**
- **3 cloves**
- **2 slices of fresh ginger**
- **Salt to taste.**
- **extra virgin olive oil as needed**

Finely chop the shallot and set it aside. Prepare the fresh ginger by cutting two rounds from the root, remove the peel, and cut them coarsely. Also, prepare the other spices required by the recipe for use. In the meantime, wash the pumpkin and cut it into medium sized pieces without removing the skin. Put the already prepared vegetable broth on the fire (even just the water is fine) and put it to heat so that it is already hot when we add it to the pumpkin. Put a saucepan with two tablespoons of extra virgin olive oil and half a coffee glass of water on the stove: add the shallot, ginger, cloves, and curry. Sauté gently for a few minutes, stirring often. At this point, add the pumpkin cut into pieces, brown it in a pot for a few seconds, add the salt and mix well. Add the vegetable broth or water until it is covered. Cook over high heat for about 20 minutes, add salt, and turn off. Remove the cloves and proceed with an immersion blender, blending the mixture until a soft and velvety cream is obtained. Serve hot with a drizzle of raw oil, a sprinkling of toasted sesame seeds, and croutons.

•Pumpkin and walnut rice salad

Ingredients:
- **100 g of cooked brown rice**
- **200 g of grated pumpkin**
- **1 apple**
- **10 walnut kernels**
- **1 handful of mustard sprouts**
- **2 tablespoons of oil**
- **1 tablespoon of wine vinegar**
- **pepper**
- **salt**

It is a recipe that lends itself to recycling previously cooked rice or other grains. Season the brown rice with crumbled walnut kernels, apart from washing and peeling an apple and pumpkin. Prepare a diced apple and pumpkin to sauté in a pan in a bit of oil and a salt pinch. Transfer the seasoning to a bowl with the rice and walnuts and season everything with oil, vinegar, and ground pepper. To close, distribute the mustard sprouts evenly.

•Autumn garden soup

Ingredients:
- **1 small leek**
- **2 cloves of minced garlic**
- **2 tablespoons of minced ginger**
- **100 g of celeriac**
- **200 g of carrots**
- **200 g of potatoes**
- **100 g of beetroot**
- **about 1 l of vegetable broth**
- **2 tablespoons of chives**
- **1 teaspoon of oil**
- **salt**

Cut the leek in half lengthwise and then into small pieces; the other diced vegetables. Sauté the leek for a few minutes in the oil with a pinch of salt over low heat; add half of the garlic and ginger, cook for a minute. Put the other vegetables in the pot and let it all flavor; then pour in the broth and a nice pinch of salt, bring to a boil and cook covered, simmering over low heat for about 30 minutes. Before serving, sprinkle with the remaining minced garlic and ginger. Garnish the individual portions of soup with finely chopped chives.

•Cream of corn

Ingredients:

- 450 g of sweet corn
- 1 small white onion
- 380 g of potatoes
- 1 teaspoon of vegetable butter
- 300 ml of vegetable broth
- 350 ml of oat milk
- 1 lime
- White pepper

To garnish

- slices of avocado
- parsley leaves

In a high-sided saucepan, soften the butter and brown the onion and peeled potatoes cut into small cubes for 5 minutes, stirring and making sure they do not burn. Then add the drained corn, the vegetable broth, and the oat milk. Bring slowly to a boil, lightly salt, and cook for 30 minutes. After this time, purée everything with a fine-texture vegetable mill, helping with the cooking liquid. The filter will only have to retain the well-pressed skins, especially those of the corn kernels. Otherwise, the flavor will be lost. Stir in the lime juice and make the cream homogeneous. Serve it in bowls decorated with a thin slice of avocado and a sprinkle of pepper; give the final touch with a leaf of parsley.

Single Course

•Vegetable crumble

Ingredients:
- **2 small zucchini**
- **2 potatoes**
- **1 leek**
- **1 pepper**
- **stale bread**
- **Origan**
- **2 cloves of garlic**
- **salt and pepper**

Preheat the oven to 250 degrees. Clean and wash the vegetables. Make a lot of cubes (the smaller the pieces, the faster they cook). Gather them in a bowl and season with salt, pepper, and a little oil. Separately, with the help of a robot, crush a few slices of bread, along with garlic and oregano. You have to get some breadcrumbs.
Transfer all the vegetables to a baking sheet and cover them with fragrant breadcrumbs. Drizzle with a drizzle of oil and bake for 15 minutes.

•Baked spaghetti

Ingredients:
- •350 g of wholemeal spaghetti
- •10 cherry tomatoes
- •1 small eggplant
- •1 cloves of garlic
- •200 g of tomato sauce
- •20 black olives
- •4 basil leaves
- •4 tablespoons of extra virgin olive oil
- •Salt to taste
- •1 chilli

Wash the eggplant, dry it and cut it into cubes. Put it in a pan with the peeled and halved garlic, the chopped chili, two tablespoons of oil, and four of water. Add salt and cook for 5 minutes over high heat, stirring occasionally. Add the tomatoes divided into four and continue cooking for the same amount of time. Complete with the sauce, the sliced olives, and the chopped basil. Boil the spaghetti in salted water for the time indicated on the package. Mix them immediately with the sauce, season with salt, and season with the remaining oil. Prepare 4 large pieces of parchment paper and distribute the spaghetti. Close the packets well and bake them at 180∞ for about 10 minutes. Transfer them to plates and serve.

•Eggplant pie

Ingredients:
- •2 large eggplants
- •2 cloves of garlic
- •800 g of large ripe tomatoes
- •1 bunch of basil
- •1 lemon
- •a few pitted green olives
- •4 tablespoons of extra virgin olive oil
- •salt and chilli to taste

Blanch the tomatoes, peel them, and cut them into pieces. Put them in a pan with 2 tablespoons of oil, minced garlic, salt, and chili. Make them thicken. In the end, season them with the remaining oil and parsley. Meanwhile, check the eggplants, wash and dry them. Cut them into slices about a couple of centimeters thick, salt them lightly and brush them with a bit of oil. Cook them on a wire rack until soft, then remove and set aside. To serve, line up a few slices of eggplant on a plate and cover with a little sauce. Overlap the others and cover with the tomato and basil, continuing in this way until all the ingredients are used up.

•Cous cous with 7 vegetables

Ingredients:
250 grams of cooked chickpeas
450 grams of cooked couscous
6 tablespoons of extra virgin olive oil
1 small onion
1 cinnamon stick
200 grams of eggplant
2 carrots
3 potatoes
150 grams of pumpkin
100 grams of green beans
2 zucchini
2 tomatoes
1 sprig of parsley
half a teaspoon of sweet paprika
half a teaspoon of cumin powder
Salt and Pepper To Taste

Chop the onion, cut the eggplants into approximately 2 cm cubes, potatoes and squash a little smaller. Carrots and zucchini in slices, green beans, and chopped tomatoes. Slowly soften the onion in the oil with the cinnamon stick in a large pot. Add carrots, eggplants, potatoes, tomatoes, and a pinch of salt; add the spices and the sprig of parsley tied with a stem of the parsley itself (it will be easier to remove it at the end of cooking), and let it flavor. Cover with boiling water and cook in a covered pot over low heat for 15 minutes. Then add the pumpkin and chickpeas and continue cooking for another 5 minutes; add the green beans and zucchini. Finish cooking and add salt if necessary.

The preparation must remain a bit soupy to season the couscous, and the vegetables must be tender but not undone.

• Risotto with radicchio and almond cream

Ingredients:
•350 grams of semi-whole rice
•1 onion
•1 leek
•200 grams of red radicchio
•1 liter of vegetable broth
•2 tablespoons of almond cream
•50 grams of flaked almonds
•salt and oil to taste

Peel and wash the radicchio, cut it into slices, and set it aside. Heat the vegetable broth and keep it warm. Cut the onion and leek into thin slices and sauté them in a saucepan with oil, salt, and 3-4 tablespoons of broth, cover and turn from time to time. Add the rice, brown it, and pour a broth ladle; cook, stirring constantly, and gradually add the broth. When there are 10 minutes left to cook, add salt and pepper to taste. Now incorporate the radicchio (set aside a little for the decoration) and cook it so that it is just crunchy, diluting the risotto with a bit of broth to keep it creamy. Remove from the heat and stir in the almond cream. Serve, garnish with fresh radicchio and a few flakes of almonds.

•Pasta with chard cream

Ingredients:
•350 g of wholemeal spelled pasta
•500 g of chard
•2 shallots
•500 g of vegan bechamel sauce
•2 tablespoons of grated Parmesan cheese
•3 tablespoons of dry white wine
•vegetable broth
•3 tablespoons of oil
•Salt to taste.

Clean the beets and separate the stems from the leaves. Wash and cut them into small pieces. Chop the shallots, put them in a pan with a tablespoon of oil and the wine. Let them soften, stirring occasionally, then add the stalks of the chard. Salt lightly. Stir briefly and sprinkle with a bit of broth. Cover and cook over low heat, adding more broth when needed. Meanwhile, wash the leaves and steam them or boil them in a pot with boiling water. Let them cool and cut them into fine strips. Mix the cooked stems and mix them with the bechamel. Add the leaves and the Parmesan. Heat the sauce, and in the meantime, boil the pasta in plenty of boiling water. Once the pasta is cooked, add it to the sauce, toss it briefly with the chard cream and serve it seasoned with the remaining oil.

•Pumpkin rice

Ingredients:
- **1 cup of brown rice**
- **1 onion**
- **400 g of clean pumpkin**
- **3 cups of vegetable broth**
- **1 sprig of rosemary**
- **3 tablespoons of oil**

Put the rice in a saucepan with 2 cups of broth. Cover and bring it to a boil, then lower the heat and cook slowly for an hour. Meanwhile, finely chop the onion and transfer it to a pan just covered with broth. Let it soften over medium heat for a few minutes before adding the diced pumpkin and rosemary leaves. Pour in the remaining broth and cook over low heat for 10-15 minutes. Add the pumpkin to the cooked rice and leave to rest for 5 minutes. Season with oil and salt, stir, and serve.

•Chickpea flans with black cabbage

Ingredients:
- **400 g of boiled and drained chickpeas**
- **500 g of black cabbage**
- **2 cloves of garlic**
- **vegetable broth**
- **2 tablespoons of lemon juice**
- **100 g of sunflower seeds**
- **60-80 g of breadcrumbs**
- **1 teaspoon of thyme**
- **salt**
- **3 tablespoons of oil**

Remove the black cabbage from the rib, wash it, and put it in a saucepan with the minced garlic. Add salt and thyme. Cook over medium heat for about ten minutes, adding a little broth when needed. In the end, let it cool and go to the mixer. Transfer the vegetables to a plate. Collect the drained chickpeas, lemon juice, sunflower seeds, and salt in a blender. Finely chop them with the help of a bit of broth. Pour everything into a bowl with three-quarters of the black cabbage. Add the breadcrumbs necessary to have a compact but still soft mixture. Grease 4 molds of the desired shape with a bit of oil. Bake at 190 degrees for 15-20 minutes. Serve the flans directly in the molds, accompanied by the cabbage, and seasoned with the remaining oil.

• Broccoli and sweet potato pie

Ingredients:
- **300 g of sweet potatoes**
- **400 g of broccoli**
- **2 cloves of garlic**
- **1 bunch of parsley**
- **1 glass of vegetable broth**
- **3 tablespoons of oil**
- **salt**

Peel and wash the sweet potatoes, then cut them into slices that are not too thick. Peel and clean the broccoli; slice the stems and divide the flowers into florets. Finely chop garlic and parsley. Line a baking sheet with parchment paper and brush it with a tablespoon of oil mixed with water. Make the first layer with the potatoes and a pinch of salt, a second with the broccoli and a little more salt, a third with garlic and parsley. Finish with the potatoes and pour over all the broth. Bake at 190 degrees for about 40 minutes. When cooked, season with the remaining oil and serve.

• Green rolls

Ingredients:
• a few leaves of Chinese cabbage (or savoy cabbage)
• 1 bunch of chard
• natural sauerkraut

Bring plenty of water to a boil, add a pinch of salt and the whole cabbage leaves; cook them until tender and let them drain. Cook the chard in the same water, leaving the leaves whole but separated from the stems, which must cook a little longer. They must maintain a bright green color. Drain them well, squeezing away the excess water. Then wrap the chard, and a sprig of sauerkraut in the cabbage leaves to make rolls. Cut each roll into two pieces.

Dessert

•Raspberry pie

Ingredients:
•2 cups of wholemeal flour
•the peel of half a lemon (preferably organic)
•1 tablespoon of rice malt
•a pinch of salt
•1 glass of water

For the filling:
•300-400 g of raspberries
•100 g of fresh ricotta

Preheat the oven to 180 degrees. In a bowl, prepare the dough for the base of the tart. Mix the grated lemon peel, a spoonful of rice malt or honey, and a pinch of salt with the flour. Dissolve the dough in water (preferably at room temperature) until it forms a firm stick of dough. With the help of a rolling pin, roll out the dough into a low cake pan, lightly greased with oil or covered with baking paper. Then bake in a hot oven (180 degrees) for 15 minutes. When the tart's bottom appears golden brown, remove it from the oven and let it cool for a few minutes. Before serving, spread the fresh ricotta on the base (it is optional to sweeten it with brown sugar or honey) and distribute the washed and delicately dried raspberries with a cloth.

•Coffee Mousse

Ingredients:
- •500 ml of rice milk
- •3 cups of coffee
- •100 g of raw cane sugar
- •100 g of rice flour

Gather the flour and sugar in a bowl; mix them well. Pour the rice milk with the coffee into a saucepan, slowly add the flour mixture and beat with a whisk until everything is well blended. Put the mixture on low heat and, still stirring, bring it to a boil. Cook it for 3-4 minutes while mixing, then pour it into a bowl and let it cool in a cold bain-marie, stirring occasionally. If lumps form, remove them with an immersion blender. Let the mousse cool in the fridge for 3-4 hours, then serve it in individual glasses or casseroles.

•Grandmother's cake

Ingredients:
- •350 g of semi-wholemeal or kamut flour
- •80 g of corn malt
- •80 ml of organic corn oil
- •10 g of fresh brewer's yeast
- •120 ml of warm water
- •1 scant teaspoon of cinnamon or vanilla in
- •powder (if you like both too)
- •the grated rind of 1 lemon
- •1 pinch of salt

Cocoa cream:
- •250 g of corn malt
- •370 ml of almond milk
- •50 g of corn starch
- •40 g of unsweetened cocoa powder
- •1 pinch of salt

Start by preparing the cocoa cream: pour 300 ml of almond milk, the malt, a pinch of salt into a pan and cook over low heat, often stirring to prevent it from sticking. Separately, in another container, combine the cornstarch and the bitter cocoa, mix well with a whisk's help, and incorporate the remaining milk: when the pot on the stove reaches the boiling point, add the starch and cocoa, and stir to prevent lumps from forming. Within a few minutes, the cream thickens, let it cool before using it to fill the cake. Prepare the dough: dissolve the brewer's yeast in warm water and let it rest. Meanwhile, in a large container, put the flour, vanilla and/or cinnamon, salt, and lemon peel, make a hole in the center and incorporate the oil as the first wet ingredient, working it with a bit of dough.

It is always starting from the center, adding the water with the yeast and malt, taking care to work well, and energetically all the ingredients together, if necessary, to help yourself with a bit of flour. Once you have obtained a homogeneous mixture, transfer it to a work surface and work it carefully with circular movements until you have an elastic and soft compound. Let it rest for 30 minutes before dividing it into two parts: 300 g, which you will use for the base, and the rest for the covering on the surface. With a rolling pin, roll out the base forming a disk of about 30 cm, arrange it on the baking sheet lined with parchment paper and press the inside corners of the pastry well with your thumbs to shape the edge. Then spread the cold cocoa cream, spreading it well. Knead the remaining dough and form a disc of about 28 cm: place it on the cake and, with the help of the tip of the handle of a spoon, tuck the edge with the one below to seal the cake. Prick the surface with a fork in various points and bake at 200 ° for 40 minutes until the pastry is golden. Remove from the oven and immediately brush with the polish, then sprinkle with coconut and bitter cocoa.

•Cocoa Puffs

Ingredients:
- **170 grams of almond flour**
- **1 liter of rice milk**
- **50 grams of raisins**
- **finely chopped almonds (or hazelnuts)**
- **50 grams of coconut flour**
- **2-3 tablespoons of rice malt**
- **1 bay leaf**
- **1 pinch of sea salt**

Bring the rice milk to a boil with the bay leaf. Add the raisins and flour and cook for 15 minutes over low heat, stirring constantly. Turn off the heat, remove the bay leaf, then add the almonds, coconut, and malt. Leave to cool. Shape into balls of 4-5 cm in diameter and roll them in coconut flour. To serve.

•Banana dessert

Ingredients:
- 50 g of pitted dates
- 10 g of sultanas
- 100 g of Pecan nuts
- 50 g of peeled almonds
- 50 g of Rapè coconut
- Himalayan salt
- 1 tablespoon of orange juice
- 1 tablespoon of coconut oil
- cinnamon powder

For the stuffing
- 2 large bananas
- 420 g of cashews soaked for about 6-7 hours
- the juice and grated zest of ½ organic lemon
- 150 ml of agave syrup, cooled in the freezer for about 25 minutes
- 150 g of cocoa butter
- 1 tablespoon of coconut oil

To garnish
- ½ bar of dark chocolate or maple syrup or chopped hazelnuts
- banana slices (optional)

Wash the dates and raisins under running water, then chop them finely in a mixer; without turning off the appliance, add the salt, orange juice, coconut oil, and cinnamon. When you have obtained a compact mixture, add the Pecan nuts and the chopped almonds in thin grains separately, complete with the Rapè coconut. Mix the dough well and roll it out on the bottom of a small cake pan (or a loaf pan), which you will have lined with baking paper. Level it well on the surface using a spatula and put it to solidify in the freezer or refrigerator. Drain the cashews and grind them for a long time in the mixer to make them doughy. Continuing to operate, first add the lemon juice and zest, agave syrup, cocoa butter, and melted coconut oil; then add the bananas and continue until you have a soft cream. Pour it on the cooled base and place it in the freezer, so that it becomes firm. You can also divide it into individual portions. Let it cool for a few minutes before serving. Decorate with a few banana slices, if you like, or with dark chocolate cut into flakes or with maple syrup and chopped hazelnuts.

•Almond and apricot cake

Ingredients:

- **500g of chopped apricots + other ripe ones for garnish**
- **½ cup of chopped dried apricots**
- **2 tablespoons of agar-agar**
- **2 cups of almond milk**
- **2 tablespoons of almond cream**
- **the grated zest of ½ lemon**
- **1 teaspoon of vanilla**
- **4 tablespoons of corn starch**
- **½ cup of concentrated apple juice**
- **200 g of ladyfingers**
- **Apple juice**
- **salt**

Put the fresh and dried apricots in a pot together with half a cup of water, the agar-agar, and a pinch of salt. Stirring constantly, bring to a boil, and cook for 5-10 minutes. When cooked, add the concentrated juice, then blend. Use a little almond milk to dissolve the corn starch and rest on the heat with a pinch of salt, lemon peel, and vanilla. When it is about to boil, remove it from the stove, add the almond cream and starch, and then let it boil again and turn it off. Blend the apricots, add the cream and adjust the flavor by adding, if necessary, more concentrated apple juice. Cut the ladyfingers at one end and quickly dip them in the apple juice. Arrange them standing along the edge of a mold of about 22 cm and distribute the cutouts on the bottom. Cover with the apricot cream and leave to cool for a few hours. Remove the hinge from the mold and serve the cake decorated with some halved fresh apricots.

•Strawberry tartlets

Ingredients:
For the shortcrust pastry
- **250 g of wholemeal flour**
- **50 g of coconut butter**
- **2 tablespoons of rice flour**
- **2 tablespoons of brown sugar**
- **1 teaspoon of ground cinnamon**
- **1 pinch of pink salt**

For coverage
- **4 tablespoons of unsweetened apricot jam**
- **2 tablespoons of chopped hazelnuts**
- **½ tablespoon of lemon juice**
- **1 tablespoon of cherry, plum or apricot distillate**
- **400 g of strawberries**
- **1 sprig of mint**

Melt the coconut butter in a double boiler and let it cool. Pour it into the mixer with the other ingredients and sugar. Operate; when large crumbs begin to form, add a few tablespoons of cold water at a time, continuing to knead the dough until it collects into a ball. Wrap it in a cloth and put it in the fridge for 30 minutes. It is using a damp brush, grease 8 molds with a diameter of 10 cm with oil. Obtain from the thinly rolled dough as many discs large enough to cover the molds' walls and the bottom. They will have to adhere everywhere. Prick the bottom with a fork. Cover each tart with a piece of parchment paper and a few dried beans. Bake at 180 degrees for 15 minutes, remove the paper and the legumes, cook them for another 5 minutes. After another ten minutes, remove them, and once cold, unmold them. Heat the jam with the distillate until it is shiny. Turn off and add the lemon juice. After a few minutes, brush part of the mixture on the bases. Wash the strawberries, dry them gently and slice them not too thin. Distribute them over the dough. Cover with the remaining jam, sprinkle the surface with the grains, and let it rest in a cool place for about an hour. Just before serving, garnish the tarts with mint leaves.

•Chocolate with avocado and orange

Ingredients:
- **200 g of pitted dates soaked for 15 minutes**
- **150 g of walnut kernels**
- **150 g of white almonds**
- **1 tablespoon of orange juice**
- **1 tablespoon of coconut oil**
- **½ teaspoon of sea salt**

For the stuffing
- **5 large ripe avocados, peeled**
- **100 g of coconut oil**
- **1 tablespoon of white almond cream**
- **50 g of melted cocoa butter**
- **the grated zest of ½ orange**
- **½ teaspoon of vanilla powder**
- **170 g of cocoa powder**
- **250 g of agave syrup**

To garnish
- **dark chocolate grains**

Soak the dates for 15 minutes. Let the maple syrup cool in the freezer for about 25 minutes. Finely grind the walnuts and almonds in the bowl of a mixer. Keep them aside. In their place, put the drained dates and purée them. Then, continuing to operate the appliance, add the salt, coconut oil, orange juice, and the previously prepared grains. When you have a compact mixture, the spread is based on a pan (or a loaf pan) lined with baking paper. Level it well with a spatula and remove it in the freezer or in the refrigerator to make it firm. Gather all the ingredients required for the filling in a mixer and start. You will need to get a well blended mixture. Pour on the solidified base and pass the cake in the refrigerator or freezer so that it hardens. Decorated with one of the proposed alternatives and served.

•Chocolate nut and almond balls

Ingredients:
- **200 g of wholemeal flour**
- **150 g of walnuts**
- **50 g of pine nuts**
- **50 g of sunflower seeds**
- **200 g of almonds**
- **50 g of flax seeds**
- **100 g of raisins**
- **100 g of dark chocolate in small pieces**
- **400 g of rice malt**
- **1 lemon**
- **1 orange**
- **6 tablespoons of brown sugar**

Soak the raisins in warm water. In the meantime, grate the peel of a lemon and an organic orange and place them in a large bowl. Add the coarsely chopped walnuts and almonds, flax seeds, sunflower seeds, and pine nuts. Stir in the flour, chocolate, and squeezed raisins and mix well with your hands. Then add the malt and continue to mix all the ingredients with energy. Lightly moisten your hands and form medium-sized balls that you will arrange quite far from each other in a baking tray lined with baking paper. Bake for about 10-12 minutes at 180 °. Let cool before serving. Excellent served accompanied by a fragrant compote of apples and spices.

• Chocolate truffles

Ingredients:
- **100 g of dark chocolate**
- **100 g of almonds**
- **50 g of hazelnuts**
- **100 g of dates**
- **50 g of bitter cocoa**

Soak the almonds in a glass jar for at least 3 hours, then add the dates and leave them for another hour. Meanwhile, heat the dark chocolate in a bain-marie. Drain and set aside the almond and date water. We combine the melted chocolate in the jar with the dried fruit and work it all with the hand blender. Incorporate the chopped hazelnuts and place them in the fridge for an hour. If the mixture is too hard, wet it with one or two tablespoons of soaking liquid. We sprinkle the cocoa on a saucer. We take small doses of the mixture and let them fall on the cocoa. We form balls and compact them well, trying to press them as much as possible. Let's put them in small bowls and skewer each ball with a wooden stick.

Creams, sauces, dressings

•Eggplants sauce

Ingredients:
- **2 medium-sized eggplants**
- **1 clove of garlic**
- **abundant basil**
- **parsley**
- **a pinch of grated lemon zest**
- **20 g of pine nuts**
- **extra virgin olive oil**
- **whole sea salt**

In a saucepan, bring lightly salted water to a boil. Meanwhile, clean, peel and divide the eggplant pulp into chunks. Blanch the eggplants for 3 minutes, then blend them until they are reduced to a smooth and homogeneous cream. Season with salt and season with oil and a small piece of lemon zest. With a mixer's help, prepare an emulsified sauce based on garlic, basil, a few parsley leaves, extra virgin olive oil, and salt. Serve the eggplant sauce with the basil emulsion and the pine nuts toasted in a pan on top.

•Ginger and avocado sauce

Ingredients:
- •2 ripe avocados
- •the juice of 1 lemon
- •1 clove of garlic
- •2 tablespoons of chopped walnuts
- •1 tablespoon of fresh grated ginger
- •1 pinch of salt
- •125 grams of plain yogurt

Peel the avocados and pit them. Mash the pulp with a fork and sprinkle it immediately with the filtered lemon juice to prevent it from blackening. Add the crushed garlic and grated ginger. Finally, gently stir in the yogurt and add salt. To speed up the timing, you can put everything in the mixer.

•Almond Butter

Ingredients:
- • 100 g of peeled almonds
- • 50 g of sunflower oil
- • 70 g of coconut milk
- • the juice of half a lemon
- • salt

Reduce the almonds to an excellent powder with a coffee grinder and pour them into a mixer. Add the salt and then the liquids, operating several times until a compact cream is obtained. This butter can be kept in the refrigerator for a few days and is excellent both for creaming risotto and pasta and other savory and sweet preparations.

•Tomato pesto with almonds and pine nuts

Ingredients:
•5 tomatoes
•1 bunch of basil
•3 cloves of garlic
•3 tablespoons of ground almonds
•2 tablespoons of pine nuts
•2 tablespoons of extra virgin olive oil
•salt and chilli to taste

Wash the tomatoes and dry them, then cut them into pieces. Rinse and dry the basil, chop it coarsely, and put it in a blender together with the peeled garlic and tomatoes. Add the salt, chili pepper according to taste and oil. Blend everything until you have a homogeneous mixture. Finally, add the chopped almonds and pine nuts separately. Stir well. This pesto is excellent for seasoning cooked cereals first of all, but it is also tasty with legumes.

•Rocket pesto

Ingredients:
•1 large bunch of rocket
•2 cloves of garlic
•3 large seeded tomatoes
•10 capers
•2 tablespoons of pine nuts
•2 tablespoons of hazelnuts
•extra virgin olive oil to taste

Wash and dry the rocket. Put all the ingredients in the mixer, excluding the oil. Work them by adding the oil slowly until you have a homogeneous mixture. Instead of pine nuts and hazelnuts you can use the equivalent amount of pistachios and walnuts.

• Spiced pumpkin jam

Ingredients:
• 1 kg of pumpkin
• 3 tablespoons of 100% malt rice
• 1 cup of almonds
• 2 teaspoons of vanilla powder
• 2 teaspoons of cinnamon
• 4 cardamom capsules
• the juice and zest of 1 grated lemon
• 2 teaspoons of agar-agar

Clean the pumpkin, cut it into small pieces and make a puree that you will cook for 15 minutes with the juice and peel of the lemon and the cardamom seeds deprived of the shell. Continue cooking for another 20-30 minutes, mixing often and skimming if necessary. Add the chopped almonds, malt, cinnamon, and vanilla powder to the mixture. Mix well and add the agar-agar that you have previously dissolved in a little water and left to rest for at least 15 minutes. Continue to cook over high heat, stirring well for another 5 minutes, then put the jam in sterilized jars.

•Zucchini pesto

Ingredients:
- **Zucchini 200 g**
- **Extra virgin olive oil 125 g**
- **Salt up to 2 g**
- **Pine nuts 30 g**
- **Parmesan to grate 60 g**
- **Basil 10 g**

Wash the zucchini, remove the ends, and chop them with the help of a grater with large holes. Place the grated zucchini in a colander, salt them lightly and let them rest for 30 minutes so that they lose the excess liquid. Then pour them into the mixer with the pine nuts and basil leaves previously cleaned with a dry cloth. Add the grated Parmesan and a part of the oil. Then turn on the mixer and blend for a few seconds. Add the rest of the oil and blend until you get a smooth cream. Transfer the mixture to a bowl and use the zucchini pesto according to your needs.

•Rocket pesto

Ingredients:
- •Rocket 100 g
- •Extra virgin olive oil 150 g
- •Pine nuts 50 g
- •Parmesan to grate 100 g
- •1 clove garlic
- •Salt up to taste

Wash the rocket very well, dry it, and put it in the cup of a mixer: also add the pine nuts, the parmesan; add the whole peeled clove of garlic and salt. At this point, add a small part of the olive oil. Begin to blend everything at low speed and add the remaining olive oil gradually until you get a well combined and fluid cream.

•Sauce at nuts

Ingredients:

- **•Walnuts 160 g (shelled and without peel)**
- **•Extra virgin olive oil 70 g**
- **•1 clove garlic**
- **•Pine nuts 20 g**
- **•Parmesan to be grated 30 g**
- **•Whole milk 160 g**
- **•Marjoram 4 g**
- **•Bread crumb 30 g**

Take a bowl with high sides and pour the breadcrumbs to which you will add the milk. Mix the crumb with the milk so that it can moisten well. When the breadcrumbs have softened, pour the bowl with the bread over a tightly meshed colander placed on a small bowl to drain the excess milk and, if necessary, press lightly with a spatula. Collect the extra milk and set aside. Now take the walnuts, then add them in a mixer with bread previously soaked in milk and pine nuts. Then add garlic, marjoram, and grated cheese. Operate the blender and gradually add the oil and the milk kept aside to make your walnut sauce more creamy and thicker. Season with salt and pepper. When you have obtained a nice homogeneous mixture, your walnut sauce will be ready to flavor dishes!

•Garlic sauce

Ingredients:
- **•Garlic 4 cloves**
- **•Peeled almonds 50 g**
- **•Extra virgin olive oil 250 ml**
- **•Parsley to chop 2 tbsp**
- **•White wine vinegar 2 tbsp**
- **•Salt up to taste**
- **•Black pepper to taste**
- **•Potatoes 80 g**

Wash the potato well and boil with all the peel in salted water; when cooked (prick it with a fork to check the cooking), drain it and let it cool. Once cold, peel it and cut it into wedges. Peel the garlic and place it in the mixer, add the peeled almonds, parsley, vinegar, potatoes, salt, and pepper and blend everything incorporating the oil a little at a time. Once a thick cream is obtained, the garlic sauce will be ready to be served with your dishes.

Chapter 5: Recipes for hyperthyroidism

Breakfast

•Carrot and raisin muffins

Ingredients:
- **250 g of carrots**
- **150 g of kamut flour**
- **150 g of corn flour**
- **2 teaspoons of cream of tartar**
- **70 ml of agave juice**
- **100-120 ml of natural apple juice with no added sugar**
- **100 ml of natural vegetable cream with no added sugar**
- **90 ml of organic sunflower oil (or extra virgin olive oil)**
- **half a teaspoon of dried ginger powder**
- **1 pinch of salt**
- **2 handfuls of raisins**

Preheat the oven to 180 degrees. Soak the raisins in water and leave them for about 15 minutes. Peel and grate the carrots in a bowl. In another bowl, combine the Kamut flour, the cornflour, the cream of tartar, the salt, and the ginger. Separately, in yet another container, pour the oil, agave, apple juice, and cream. Beat with a whisk and add the liquid mixture to the flours.

 Mix and incorporate the grated carrots and raisins. Mix the dough. Pour the mixture into the muffin molds using a spoon. Bake and cook for 45-50 minutes or until the surface is slightly colored and the inside is dry enough. Remove from the oven, transfer to a wire rack, and cool for about 5 minutes before unmolding.

•Kamut cookies

Ingredients:
•500 g of kamut flour
•200 g of corn malt
•100 ml of corn oil
•200 ml of warm water
•50 g of grated coconut
•20 g of baking powder for cakes
•5 g of salt

Put the dry ingredients in a container: flour, coconut, yeast, salt, and; mix them well. Mix the malt, oil, and warm water, pour it all over the dry ingredients, and work with one hand in a circular direction, mixing the mixture well. Flour the work surface, place the dough on it and continue to knead until you get a homogeneous, soft, and elastic dough (add a little water if necessary). After a few minutes, roll out a sheet of about 1 cm thick sheet with a rolling pin, then form many biscuits with a pastry cutter or knife. Knead the leftover scraps and create other biscuits until the dough is finished. Put the biscuits in the pan and bake them in the preheated oven at 195 ° for

about 15 minutes or until they are golden. Let them cool
and serve them.

•Brioche with orange carrots and coconut

Ingredients:
•200 g of rice flour
•150 g of corn flour
•170 g of maple syrup
**•200 g of carrots already cleaned and cut into
chunks**
•100 ml of orange juice
•100 g of grated coconut
•70 g lightly toasted sunflower seeds
•70 ml of sunflower oil
•70 ml of water
25 g of cream of tartar
•the grated peel of 1 orange
•1 pinch of salt

Put the carrots in the jar of the food processor with the
salt and the grated orange peel. Start grinding, then add
the sunflower seeds and continue. Finally, add the oil,
orange juice, lo maple syrup and continue until the
mixture is well blended. Put the rice flour, cornflour,
coconut flour, and yeast in a bowl, mix well with your
hands, and then add the mixture in the mixer and the
water. Mix until you get a soft dough: lifting a little dough
with one hand and letting it go, it must fall slowly. With
the pastry bag or with a spoon, fill three-quarters of the
molds with the dough and bake in a preheated oven at
200 ° for 25 minutes. As soon as they are baked, let them
cool before serving.

•Budwig cream

Ingredients:
•3 tablespoons of soy yogurt
•½ lemon
•2 teaspoons of oil
•2 tsp flax seeds
•2 tsp raw whole grains (oats, rice, barley, buckwheat, etc.)
•1 tablespoon of rice malt

Add to the yogurt the juice of half a lemon, two teaspoons of oil, two teaspoons of flax seeds, and two teaspoons of freshly ground organic whole grains of your choice: oats, rice, barley, buckwheat, etc. add rice or barley malt.

Salty muffin

Ingredients:
- **130 g of wholemeal flour**
- **120 g of corn flour**
- **1 small carrot**
- **1 piece of leek (the green part)**
- **soya milk**
- **3 tablespoons of oil**
- **1 teaspoon of oregano**
- **3 tablespoon of mixed pumpkin, flax and sunflower seeds**
- **1 sachet of yeast**
- **salt**

Chop the seeds and put them in a bowl. Combine the two flours, oregano, yeast, and salt. Pour in the oil first, then gradually add enough milk to have a soft mixture (about 1 glass). Complete with the diced carrot and the washed and thinly sliced leek. Pour the mixture into a tall, narrow mold lined with baking paper. Bake at 180 degrees for 35-40 minutes. When cooked, allow the muffin to cool, turn it out of the mold and let it cool. Serve with a thick tomato sauce or with chopped and sautéed leeks and carrots.

•Lentil crepes

Ingredients:
- **100-120 of cooked and well dried lentils**
- **3 tablespoons of flour**
- **100-120 ml of oat milk**
- **salt**
- **oil**

For the filling:
- **tomato sauce**

Dilute the flour in the vegetable milk. Add salt and gradually pour the mixture over the lentils. Mix well. Heat a small non-stick pan with a thin layer of oil and pour half of the dough at a time. Cook each crepe on both sides for a few minutes until it is golden brown. Serve the pancakes hot, sprinkled with a drizzle of oil.

•Gluten-free pancakes

Ingredients:

•220 g of soy milk

•1 tsp apple cider vinegar

•15 g of seed oil

•1/4 vanilla bean or 1 teaspoon vanilla extract (optional)

•80 g of buckwheat flour

•40 g of rice flour

•25 g of corn starch or potato starch

•4 g of baking powder

•15 g of whole cane sugar

•a pinch of salt

•oil to oil the pan

TO SERVE

•Maple syrup

•raspberries or other fresh fruit to taste

To prepare gluten-free pancakes in a bowl, combine the soy milk, vinegar, seed oil, and vanilla. Stir and let it rest. Separately, sift the flours with the starch and yeast. Add the sugar and a pinch of salt. Mix the flours with a whisk, and then pour the liquid mixture. Stir vigorously until the dough is smooth and without lumps. Heat a non-stick pan over medium-high heat and cover the surface with a few drops of oil. When the pan is hot, pour 2 tablespoons of mixture for each pancake. When bubbles form on the surface, and the edges darken, flip the pancakes and cook the other side. Repeat the process until the dough is used up, ensuring that the pan does not get too hot. If so, remove the pan from the heat for a minute. Serve the gluten-free pancakes hot with 2-3 teaspoons of maple syrup and fresh fruit to taste.

•Donut with carob flour

Ingredients:
- **340 g of water**
- **90 g extra virgin olive oil**
- **320 g wholemeal flour**
- **70 g carob flour**
- **50 g of corn starch**
- **1 sachet of gluten-free yeast**
- **9 dates and 9 plums**
- **90 g 92% dark chocolate**
- **1 pinch of salt**

Sift the flour, carob flour, yeast, corn starch, and salt. Separately, blend the dates and plums with 140 g of water. Emulsify this mixture with the rest of the water and the oil. Combine the dry ingredients and create a soft dough. Cut the dark chocolate with a knife and add to the dough. Bake for about 40 minutes at 180 degrees.

•Radicchio and carrot muffins

Ingredients:
- **250 g of wholemeal flour**
- **1 carrot**
- **½ head of radicchio**
- **½ sachet of cream of tartar**
- **150 g of oat milk**
- **4 tablespoons of oil**
- **1-2 tablespoons of toasted linseed and sesame**
- **50 g of roasted peanuts**
- **1 pinch of salt**

Clean the radicchio, wash it and dry it, then cut it into thin slices. Wash the carrot and dry it, remove the ends and grate it. Gather the vegetables, seeds, and peanuts in a bowl. Separately, mix the flour with salt and yeast. Then add it to the bowl's contents, mix and gradually pour the milk and oil until you have a soft and creamy mixture. If it is too dry, add a little more oat milk. Pour the mixture into the appropriate cups and bake at 180 ° C for about 20 minutes. Serve the muffins warm or cold.

•Wholemeal bread croutons with soy, figs and chocolate

Ingredients:
- **1 slice of wholemeal bread**
- **soy sauce**
- **1 dried fig**
- **dark chocolate**
- **Maple syrup**

Lightly toast the bread. Then spread it with an amount of soy as you like. Spread the fig cut into small pieces or slices on top. Sprinkle with maple syrup and complete with the chopped dark chocolate. Eat immediately.

Appetizer, Snack, Side dishes

•Tofu and carrot skewers

Ingredients:
- **200 g of tofu**
- **4 slightly large carrots**
- **salt**
- **oil**
- **soy sauce**

Sear the tofu and carrots, diced in salted water. Prepare an emulsion made with two tablespoons of oil and one of soy sauce. Brush the cubes with the emulsion, and put them on the skewers alternately. Sprinkle with a pinch of salt. Bake in a scorching oven for ten minutes and enjoy the crispy skewers.

•Millet croquettes with seitan ragout

Ingredients:
- **300 g of millet**
- **100 g of red lentils**
- **900 ml of water**

For the seitan sauce
- **800 g of fresh seitan**
- **250 g of tomato pulp**
- **100 ml of red wine**
- **50 g of dried mushrooms**
- **3 tablespoons of oil**
- **1 onion**
- **1 carrot**
- **1 stick of celery**
- **salt**

Soak the mushrooms for 30 minutes, then squeeze and chop them. Brown finely chopped onion, carrot, and celery in a pan with oil. Add the seitan and cook over medium heat for 10 minutes. Add the wine and after it has evaporated, add the tomato and mushrooms. Add salt and continue cooking over low heat for about 1 hour, stirring. Wash the millet and lentils. Drain and put them in a pot with water and salt. When it boils, reduce it to a minimum. Cover and cook without stirring for 20-25 minutes. Let it cool and if it is too soft, add some breadcrumbs and let it cool completely. Form many meatballs that you will put in a pan and cook in the oven at 200 ° for 15-20 minutes. Serve the hot croquettes covered with the ragout.

•Red onions in balsamic vinegar with plums

Ingredients:
•6-7 red onions, peeled and finely chopped
•5-6 tablespoons of extra virgin olive oil
•2 tablespoons of soy sauce
•About 100 ml of hot water
•3-4 tablespoons of balsamic vinegar
•2 tablespoons of rice malt
•6-7 dried plums cut into small pieces

Soak the plums for 20-25 minutes in warm water, rinse them, cook them in boiling water for about 10 minutes, and then pass them under cold running water and drain well. Heat the oil with the soy sauce over high heat in a large pan and sauté the onions. Add the water, lower the heat and continue cooking until the bottom has dried, stirring often. Mix the balsamic vinegar and malt in a glass, add them to the onions, add the plums and cook for a few minutes before serving.

•Tofu and vegetable roll

Ingredients:
- tofu 250 g
- 1 carrot
- ¼ of cabbage
- 1 onion
- a pinch of cumin seeds (optional)
- soy sauce
- extra virgin olive oil
- salt

Boil some water where you can, then place a steaming basket on top. Thoroughly peel and wash the vegetables. With the help of a robot, finely chop the onion and apart from the carrot. First, stew the onion in a pan with a pinch of salt and then the carrot, finally adds the savoy cabbage cut into strips. In a covered pot, sauté the vegetables for 5 minutes. With the help of a fork, crush the tofu to combine with the stewed vegetables. Adjust the sauce with soy sauce and a pinch of cumin seeds. Place the dough in a damp cloth. Roll it up like a salami, tying the ends with a string to make it tightly closed and compact. Steam it for 10 minutes. When it is cold, remove it from the towel and serve it sliced, accompanied with a grain of cereal.

•Avocado bowls

Ingredients:
•200 grams of brown rice
•4 tomatoes
•4 avocados
•the juice of 2 lemons
•1 cup of vegan mayonnaise
•a small bunch of parsley
•Salt to taste

Boil the rice in a saucepan with 500 ml of cold water. Put the lid on, lower the heat to the boil and cook until the liquid is used (40-50 minutes). Transfer it to a salad bowl and let it cool. Finely chop the parsley after washing and drying it. Wash the tomatoes and cut them into cubes, then add them to the rice. Separately, mix the mayonnaise and half the lemon juice, and almost all the parsley. Add this sauce to the rice, lightly salt, and stir carefully. Peel the avocados and pit them, sprinkling them immediately with the remaining lemon juice. With the help of a teaspoon, hollow out some of the pulp to form small cups. Mix the removed pulp with the contents of the bowl. Distribute the rice in the bowls, decorate with the remaining parsley and serve.

•Vegetable puddings

Ingredients:
- **100 g of chard**
- **200 g of tofu**
- **1 handful of parsley**
- **half a cup of olives**
- **2 tablespoons of capers**
- **6 dried cherry tomatoes**
- **1 tablespoon of soy sauce**
- **half a lemon**
- **4 tablespoons of extra virgin olive oil**
- **Salt to taste**

Clean and wash the chard well. Boil it in abundant salted water for a few minutes, then drain it, leaving the shape of the leaf intact. Take four pudding molds, grease them with oil and adhere the leaves to the inner surface, protruding well beyond the edge so that once filled, you can seal the puddings. Take the tofu and blanch it for a few minutes in salted water, drain it and put it in the blender together with the parsley, capers, olives, dried tomatoes, squeezed lemon and oil. Blend well, reducing the ingredients to a compact and homogeneous cream, if necessary help yourself with a little water from cooking the tofu during this operation. Pour the mixture into each mold and seal the surface well with the edges sticking out. Put the puddings on a tray to store in the fridge, placing each pudding on top a weight in order to compact them well (for example a coffee cup filled with water). Let them rest in the fridge for about an hour before serving.

•Vegetable snacks in tofu cream

Ingredients:
•8 radishes
•2 stalks of celery
•1 carrot
•4 lettuce leaves

For the tofu cream:
•150 g of tofu
•3 tablespoons of apple cider vinegar
•1 tablespoon of extra virgin olive oil
•1 sprig of thyme
•Salt to taste.

Carefully wash the vegetables, letting the excess water drain for a few minutes. Divide the radishes in half, cut the celery stalks into chunks, and the carrots into slices. Lettuce leaves, on the other hand, should be kept whole. Blend the tofu with apple cider vinegar, oil, and salt. Fill a pastry bag with the tofu cream and decorate the vegetables to taste. With lettuce, it is possible to prepare stuffed rolls, stuffing and rolling each leaf, stopping it with a toothpick. Serve the appetizers garnished with some thyme leaves.

•Puffed rice snack

Ingredients:
•60 grams of puffed rice
•50 grams of white almonds
•50 grams of hazelnuts
•30 grams of sesame
•30 grams of raisins
•4 tablespoons of rice malt

Toast the rice in a pan over medium heat for almost 5 minutes, stirring constantly. Transfer it to a bowl. In its place, put the sesame (washed and well drained) and repeat the operation until it becomes swollen. Toast the almonds in the oven for 15 minutes at about 130 °. Do the same with the hazelnuts, and as soon as they have cooled, remove the peel. Coarsely chop the dried fruit, mix it with the rice in the bowl, and add the raisins. Heat the malt in a bain-marie, and when it is fluid, pour it over the ingredients in the bowl, pouring the sesame. Mix well, and with just moistened hands, distribute the mixture into 4 cm diameter cups. Put the sweets in a preheated oven at 180 ° for 10 minutes, making sure they do not burn. Once cooled, they will be crunchy. They keep well in a tin box for up to a week.

•Lemon tofu crepes

Ingredients:
•200 g of tofu
•1 lemon
•1 medium sized onion
•salt and oil to taste
•2 tablespoons of spelled flour for each crepe
•some fresh mint leaves
•water q.s.

Brown the finely chopped onion and, when golden brown, sauté the crumbled tofu. Leave to flavor before adding a pinch of salt and the lemon juice diluted in half a glass of water. Simmer in a half-covered pot. Once cooked, with the heat off, grate the lemon peel. For the crepes' preparation: dilute the flour and salt with the mint decoction (bring the water to a boil with a few mint leaves, then turn off) until fluid, but the dense and homogeneous mixture is obtained. Then pour half a ladle of batter on a frying pan lightly brushed with oil and boiling. Cook the crepe over high heat for 20 seconds on both sides, and turn over. Then proceed with the rest of the dough. Stuff the crepes and serve them.

•Black and white sesame crackers

Ingredients:
- •50 g of black sesame
- •50 g of white sesame
- •30 g of wholemeal flour
- •40 g of water
- •extra virgin olive oil to taste
- •Salt to taste.

Put the black and white sesame in a bowl; add half the flour, a pinch of salt, and mix. Then pour a teaspoon of oil, water, and mix. Place a sheet of parchment paper on the work surface; distribute the mixture. Overlap a second sheet and pass the rolling pin through it, pushing it lengthwise, possibly until you get a layer as high as the thickness of the seeds. Transfer to a plate and bake for 5-6 minutes; then take it out of the oven, gently pull the paper off the surface and engrave the sheet still soft with a wheel to divide it into long and narrow two-tone rectangles. Bake for another 12-15 minutes. Remove and let it cool completely; remove from the base with a spatula and separate the crackers gently with your hands.

Soups and salads

•Cream of zucchini and avocado with coriander

Ingredients:
- **800 g of small fresh zucchini**
- **1 shallot**
- **1 ½ avocado**
- **1 lemon**
- **2 tablespoons of oil**
- **extra virgin olive oil**
- **350 ml of vegetable broth**
- **fresh cilantro**
- **2 tablespoons of oil**
- **extra virgin olive oil**
- **pinch salt**

Wash the zucchini, trim them, and cut them into rings. Peel the shallot and chop it. Gather the two ingredients in a saucepan in which you have heated the oil. Let it cook for a few minutes, stirring. Then sprinkle with the vegetable broth, add salt and bring to a boil over low heat. Cook for 20 minutes. Now add tiny fresh coriander leaves, rinsed and chopped. Mix everything with the hand blender until the mixture is smooth and homogeneous. Reduce to a puree, add the peeled and pitted avocado with the lemon juice and salt. Incorporate it into the previously prepared cream, now lukewarm. Serve the soup in bowls and garnish with and other coriander leaves.

•Millet with broccoli and cauliflower

Ingredients:
- **650 g of cooked millet**
- **1 spring onion**
- **1 carrot**
- **1 head of broccoli**
- **a few florets of cauliflower**
- **1 handful of lightly toasted sunflower seeds**
- **1-2 tablespoons of oil, salt**

Finely cut spring onion and carrots; blanch broccoli and cauliflower divided into small inflorescences, in lightly salted boiling water, separately and for a few minutes. In a large pan, sauté the onion in the oil for a minute, then add the carrot and sauté until it begins to soften, add salt. Put the millet in a pan and let the flavors blend, finally add the remaining vegetables and seeds, mix well and serve.

• Spelled and bean soup

Ingredients:
- **200 g of spelled**
- **150 g of white cannellini beans**
- **1 carrot**
- **1 onion**
- **2 sticks of celery**
- **½ l of vegetable broth**
- **2 tablespoons of oil**
- **1 bay leaf**
- **salt**

Soak the beans for 8 hours. In a terracotta pot, season the chopped onion in a bit of water for a few minutes, then add the carrot and celery cut into small pieces. Add the bay leaves, beans, and rinsed spelled to the herbs. Cover them with the vegetable broth obtained using the granular vegetable cube and cook everything in a covered pot over low heat for about an hour. Serve the spelled with cannellini beans with a drizzle of extra virgin olive oil.

•Onion soup

Ingredients:
- **400 g of onions**
- **6 slices of wholemeal bread**
- **25 g of wholemeal flour**
- **4 cl of oil**
- **1 pinch of nutmeg**
- **salt**
- **pepper**

Toast the flour in a steel pan. Finely slice the onions and sauté them gently with 1 tablespoon of oil and water. Dilute the flour in 1 liter of water, add the softened onions, a pinch of salt and pepper and cook over low heat for 30 minutes. Meanwhile in the oven, lightly toast the bread. Pour the soup into a baking dish, add 3 tablespoons of oil and sprinkle with the chopped toast. Bake at 180 degrees for a few minutes using the grill to get a crust. Serve very hot sprinkled with a pinch of nutmeg.

• Cold cream of carrots with lemon

Ingredients:
- **600 g of carrots**
- **450 g of red peppers**
- **500 g of ripe tomatoes**
- **4 tablespoons of oil**
- **extra virgin olive oil**
- **1 lemon**
- **1 radish**
- **fresh mint**
- **salt**

Wash the peppers, halve them and peel them; Bake them on a baking sheet covered with parchment paper for about 30 minutes at 160 °, until the skin is covered with bubbles and turns brown. Remove them and put them in a paper bag so that they cool while remaining moist. Clean the carrots and cut them into slices. Pour them into a pot with a liter of water to a boil and cook for at least 10 minutes. Drain and set aside the cooking liquid. Mix the carrots until you get a puree. Add the peeled tomatoes, seeded and cut into chunks, peeled peppers divided into strips, lemon juice, extra virgin olive oil, and salt. Start the mixer again and, if necessary, dilute the mixture with a little of the cooking water from the vegetables to make it smooth. Pour the cream into small bowls and garnish with slices of radish and mint leaves; serve it at room temperature or after having cooled it for a couple of hours in the refrigerator.

•Cold cream of zucchini

Ingredients:
• ½ white onion, peeled and cut into small
pieces
• 3-4 medium zucchini, cleaned and cut into
rings
• about 300 ml of vegetable broth
• 1 generous handful of fresh, clean basil
• 5-6 tablespoons of extra virgin olive oil
• 1 pinch of salt

Heat the oil over medium heat in a saucepan and sauté
the onion. Add the zucchini, salt and cook for 10 minutes,
stirring often. Remove from heat and puree everything
briefly with an immersion blender or traditional mixer.
Add the basil to the zucchini and blend again until you get
a smooth cream. Let it cool first at room temperature and
then in the refrigerator. When it is cold, arrange the soup
in individual bowls or plates, complete with a drizzle of
oil, and a few basil leaves, and serve.

• Chickpea salad

Ingredients:
- **2 cups of cooked chickpeas**
- **1 carrot**
- **10 of dried tomatoes in oil**
- **1 sprig of mint leaves**
- **1 tuft of parsley leaves**
- **1 handful of basil leaves**
- **juice and peel of ½ lemon**
- **2 tablespoons of oil**
- **salt**

After cooking the chickpeas in a pot with plenty of water, cut the carrots into thin slices, chop the aromatic herbs and cut the dried tomatoes into very thin strips. To prepare the dressing in a bowl, mix the lemon juice, lemon peel, and oil; mix well. Put all the salad ingredients in a bowl and pour the dressing. Mix well and serve.

•Cream of celery

Ingredients:
- **700 g of celery**
- **1 onion**
- **1 leek**
- **2 medium potatoes**
- **1 liter of vegetable broth**
- **1 bay leaf**
- **1 teaspoon of thyme**
- **2 tablespoons of extra virgin olive oil**
- **salt**

Chop the onion, leek, and celery. Put them in a saucepan and cover them with the broth. Let them soften over low heat for about 10 minutes, stirring often. Add the peeled and diced potatoes and pour the remaining broth along with the thyme and bay leaf. When it boils, lower the heat and cook for 20 minutes. Remove the bay leaf and puree the soup with an immersion blender. Season with salt, season with oil, and serve hot.

•Onion and oat cream with saffron

Ingredients:
•6 tablespoons of oil
•3 golden onions
•pinch salt
•About 1 liter of water
•100 g of oat flakes
•300 ml of natural oat milk with no added sugar
•1 sachet of saffron powder

Heat 4-5 tablespoons of extra virgin olive oil in a saucepan and sauté the onions, cleaned and cut into slices, over high heat. Salt, add the water, lower the heat, and cover. Soak the oat flakes in 80-100 ml of filtered water and set aside. Continue cooking the onion until tender, then add the soaked oat flakes, oat milk, and saffron, dissolved in a little hot filtered water. Cook for another 10-15 minutes, stirring often. Turn off the heat, blend the soup with an immersion blender, possibly adding more oat milk if you prefer an even finer cream.

•Cream of pumpkin soup with curry croutons

Ingredients
•About 1 kg of sweet pumpkin
•1 onion
•3 bay leaves
•1 spoon of barley or rice miso
•parsley to taste
•5 slices bread
•oil to taste
•Salt to taste.

Peel the pumpkin and cut it into small pieces. Cut the onion into cubes, p in a saucepan wither the onion with a nice pinch of salt for a few minutes with a bit of oil. Add the pumpkin, bay leaf, and water until just covering everything. Cook covered for about 15-20 minutes, until tender. Remove the bay leaves, and pass the rest with a vegetable mill. Thus, put the cream back on the heat and add the miso diluted with a bit of hot broth, simmer gently for a couple of minutes. Toast the diced bread in the oven with a bit of oil, and salt. Serve the soup with the chopped parsley and croutons.

Single course

•Fennel and bean pie

Ingredients:
• the outer leaves of 8 fennel (including the green part)
• 400 g of boiled beans
• 4 slices of stale bread
• 1 bay leaf
• 4 sprigs of thyme
• 4 parsley stalks
• 2 lemons
• 1 tablespoon of coriander seeds
• 3 tablespoons of oil
• salt

Blanch the already washed fennel. Drain and let them cool, then cut them into strips. Put them in a saucepan. Add 500 ml of the cooking water (if this is not enough, lengthen it), oil, lemon juice, salt, coarsely pounded whole pimento and coriander, aromatic herbs. Simmer them for 10-15 minutes until they are soft and the liquid has evaporated. Eliminate the laurel. Blend the beans with the help of a bit of cooking water: you must have a fairly soft mixture. Season it with salt and mix it with the beans. Complete with the bread cut into cubes (it will absorb the liquid). Put the mixture in a mold moistened with water and press it well. Turn it out on a serving plate. Wash and chop the green twigs of the fennel and distribute them on the pie.

•Barley and rice with ginger-scented asparagus

Ingredients:
- **220 g of hulled barley**
- **50 g of wild rice**
- **500 g of asparagus**
- **1 piece of ginger (3 cm)**
- **3 tablespoons of oil**
- **salt**

Wash the barley, drain it and soak it (1 cup of barley - 3 cups of water) for about 8 hours. Wash the rice, drain it and transfer everything to the pot with the barley and its soaking water. Cook in a pot for 45 minutes. Meanwhile, peel the asparagus and thinly slice the stem, leaving the tips whole. Cut half of the ginger root into thin threads and grate the rest to squeeze two juice tablespoons. In a pan, heat the oil and sauté the strands of ginger over high heat until they turn golden, then add the asparagus stems and a pinch of salt. Cook for a couple of minutes, then add the tips as well, continuing to mix. The asparagus must remain crunchy and bright in color. Add the cereals, drizzle with ginger juice, mix and serve immediately.

•Tart of peppers with tomato

Ingredients:
- •4 large yellow peppers
- •400 g of tomatoes
- •3 tablespoons of extra virgin olive oil
- •a few basil leaves
- •salt

For the dough:
- •200 g of wholemeal flour
- •30 ml of extra virgin olive oil
- •30 g of toasted sesame seeds
- •8 g of fresh brewer's yeast
- •1 pinch of salt
- •1 teaspoon of malt
- •100 ml of warm water

Start by preparing the dough: dissolve the yeast and malt in the water; let it rest for 5-7 minutes. Incorporate the other ingredients and knead them, forming an elastic and smooth dough into a ball. Let it rest for 1 hour covered. Peel the peppers, wash them, halve them and put them in the oven at 220 ° for 15 minutes; peel them and cut them into strips. Blanch the tomatoes, peel and chop them. In a pan, pour a drizzle of oil and cook the tomatoes, ½ ladle of water, basil, salt, cover, and finish cooking for 15 minutes over low heat. Let it cool down. Roll out the dough into a 30 cm disc. Arrange it on the pan; shape the edge with your thumbs, and distribute the cold filling. Bake at 190 degrees for 25-30 minutes. Serve the tart hot or warm.

•Buckwheat flan and red lentils

Ingredients:
- **350 g of buckwheat**
- **700 ml of hot vegetable broth**
- **300 g of red lentils**
- **300 ml of water**
- **2 onions**
- **3 tablespoons of oil**
- **1 teaspoon of thyme**
- **Salt to taste**
- **1 chilli**
- **50 g of sunflower seeds**
- **1 tablespoon of soy sauce**

Cook the chopped onions and chili in a pan with a bit of oil for 2 minutes. Add the red lentils, water, thyme, and salt, cover, and bring to a boil. Lower to low and cook until all the water is absorbed. Toast the sunflower seeds for 15 minutes in a preheated oven at 170 °. Immediately transfer them to a bowl with the soy sauce and stir until they have absorbed it. Wash the buckwheat, drain well, and heat it in a saucepan greased with oil; add the broth and bring to a boil. Lower to the minimum, add salt, put the lid on, and cook without stirring for 20 minutes or until the water is absorbed. Finally, add the red lentil mixture, stir, cover and continue cooking for 2 minutes. Transfer to the pan, level, and bake at 200 ° for 25-30 minutes. Remove from the oven, let it cool for a few minutes, turn over on a serving dish and remove the parchment paper. Sprinkle the sunflower seeds and serve immediately.

•Tofu, Swiss chard and carrot plumcake

Ingredients:
- **500 g of tofu**
- **500 g of chard (or spinach)**
- **300 g of carrots**
- **300 g of pumpkin**
- **extra virgin olive oil to taste**
- **Salt to taste.**

Wash the chard and blanch for 2 minutes in boiling water with a pinch of salt; drain and squeeze them very well (if you use spinach, it will be enough to put them in a pot without completely draining them or adding liquid, and cook them covered for a few minutes). Cut the carrots into rings and the pumpkin into pieces. Steam them separately, or, always separately, with a drop of oil and stew them with a pinch of salt and very little water. In this way the vegetables will be tastier, the important thing is that they are dry after cooking. Reduce them to a puree with a blender: season the chard with oil, salt, and nutmeg; carrots with oil, salt, and coriander; pumpkin with oil, salt, and cinnamon. Pass the tofu to the mixer and divide it into three equal parts; mix them respectively with the spinach, carrot, and pumpkin cream, checking their flavor. Line a loaf pan with wet and squeezed baking paper; Transfer the mixture with the pumpkin, the one with the spinach, and the one with carrots in order. Level and place in a convection oven at 180 ° for about 40 minutes. Let it cool and gently unmold.

•Vegetable paella with seitan

Ingredients:
- **300 grams of brown rice**
- **100 grams of seitan**
- **10 broccoli (or cauliflower)**
- **3 tablespoons of fresh peas**
- **1 onion**
- **1 carrot**
- **2 liters of cooking water for the vegetables**
- **1 teaspoon of saffron powder**
- **2 tablespoons of extra virgin olive oil**
- **Salt to taste**

Boil the peas and broccoli in a pot full of water and set them aside (do not throw away the water). Heat the oil in a low and wide pan, put the sliced onion and brown it, then add the chopped carrot and, after a couple of minutes, the rice and sauté for 2 or 3 minutes. Add the seitan cut into bite-sized pieces, the water kept aside, and melt the saffron. Taste and add salt. Cook uncovered and over medium heat until all the liquid is absorbed. Check the cooking and, if necessary, add a little more hot liquid. Pour in the broccoli and peas at this point. Mix well and serve

•Spelled with mushrooms and pumpkin

Ingredients:
•250 grams of pearl spelled
•700 ml of water
•1 onion
•20 grams of mushrooms
•300 grams of pumpkin
•Salt to taste.
•extra virgin olive oil to taste
•a sprig of chopped parsley

Soak the mushrooms for 30 minutes in warm water, squeeze and slice them thin; keep the soaking water aside after filtering it. Dice the onion and pumpkin. Peel the pumpkin, and cut them into small pieces. Season the onion in two tablespoons of oil, stirring for a few minutes; when they are wilted, add the pumpkin and simmer for 5 minutes. Then add the mushrooms and spelled, add the water (including the soaking water) and add salt. Cook for 30-40 minutes over low heat and with a lid. When the spelled is ready, add a drizzle of oil and mix. Garnish with plenty of chopped parsley and serve hot.

•Pasta with turnip and pine nuts

Ingredients:
•350 grams of short pasta
•300 grams of turnip greens
•1 clove of garlic
•2 handfuls of raisins
•2 handfuls of pine nuts (unsalted)
•5 tablespoons of extra virgin olive oil
•Salt to taste.
•1 pinch of red pepper

Put the raisins in warm water. Clean the turnip greens by removing the hardest and most fibrous parts of the stems. Cut into small pieces. Bring plenty of salted water to a boil, add the vegetables and when the boil resumes, immerse the pasta as well. Meanwhile, brown the minced garlic clove in oil; add the pine nuts, the drained raisins and the chilli pepper, leave to flavor. Drain the pasta, pour them into the pan and mix. Drizzle each portion with a drizzle of oil.

•Millet with pesto and tomato sauce

Ingredients:
- **350 g of millet**
- **150 g of basil pesto**
- **120 g of fresh ripe tomatoes**
- **3 spring onions**
- **salt**

Lightly toast the millet in a saucepan. Then cook it in water for about 20 minutes. Meanwhile, in a bowl, gather the tomatoes cut into small pieces and reduce them to the sauce with an immersion blender. Towards the end of cooking the millet, add the tomato sauce, stir, and heat. Clean and slice the spring onions, and add them to a bowl together with the pesto. Mix well. Add the millet with the sauce, combine it with the pesto and the rest of the ingredients, season with salt and serve immediately.

•Vegetable burger with tofu

Ingredients:
•250 g of steamed carrots
170 g of tofu
•170 g of medium-grain couscous
•170 ml of vegetable broth
•chickpea flour
•3 tablespoons of oil
•salt

Heat the broth and pour it over the couscous; salty. Stir and let it swell for 10 minutes, then transfer to a mixer with the chopped carrots and tofu and the oil. Blend and compact the mixture with a bit of chickpea flour. Take it a little at a time with wet hands and form mini-burgers which you will place on a baking sheet lined with baking paper and brushed with the remaining oil. Bake the meatballs at 190 ° for about 20 minutes, turning them once gently. Serve

Dessert

•**Cake with strawberries and coconut**

Ingredients for the base:
* 150 g of toasted soy flakes
* 150 g of oat flakes
* 50 g of whole cane sugar
* 60 g of coconut oil

Ingredients for the cream:
* 400 g of silken tofu
* 250 g of coconut cream
* 50 g of whole cane sugar
* 6 g of agar-agar
* 200 g of strawberries

First, prepare the cake base, blending the soy and oat flakes with the brown sugar. Transfer everything to a bowl and mix in the coconut oil previously dissolved in a bain-marie. Transfer the mixture obtained to a 26 cm diameter opening pan, leveling it very well, then put it in the refrigerator to harden (at least a couple of hours). Remember, at this point in the recipe, to put the coconut cream in the fridge. When the base is well hardened, it is time for the cream to separate the liquid part of the coconut cream, pour it into a glass, and keep it aside. Whip the fat part with a whisk. Stir in the silky tofu blended with the sugar, mixing with a spatula, and then the agar-agar dissolved in the coconut water kept aside. Blend for a few seconds and spread the cream evenly on the cooled base. Place the cake in the refrigerator for about an hour until the cream has solidified.

At this point, completely cover the cake with the sliced strawberries and put it back again so that it cools down for at least one night.

•Sweet coconut and cocoa

Ingredients:
- **200 g of wholemeal flour**
- **100 g of cocoa**
- **the grated zest of 1 orange**
- **100 g of brown sugar**
- **250 ml of coconut milk**
- **100 g of raisins**
- **50 g of pine nuts**
- **1 c of cream of tartar**

Soak the raisins for 15 minutes in hot water. Mix the flour with the cocoa, the cream of tartar, the orange peel, the sugar, and the cinnamon. Gradually add the coconut milk without stopping stirring, then add the squeezed raisins and finally the pine nuts. Line a round mold with baking paper. Turn the mixture over and level it well on the surface. Bake at 190 degrees for about 25 minutes. When cooked, let the cake cool.

• Oat flake cake

Ingredients:
- **250 g of oat flakes**
- **120 g of type 1 flour**
- **50 g of coconut**
- **180 g of rice malt**
- **75 ml of deodorized sunflower oil**
- **300 g of prunes or dried apricots**
- **1 lemon**
- **salt**

Soak the dried fruit in water for a few hours and then cook it with a pinch of salt until it becomes soft; make a cream of it, undoing it with a spoon, and flavor it with the grated rind of the lemon. Gather the flakes in a large bowl with the flour, salt, and coconut. Add the oil and the malt mixed in another container and mix everything. Grease a pan and distribute half of the dough, pressing it with your hands; sprinkle it with the dried fruit cream and cover carefully with the rest of the dough. Bake at 200 ° for about 50 minutes or until golden brown. To enjoy it better, let the cake cool for a few hours.

•Berries tart

Ingredients for the tart:
- **230 g of wholemeal flour**
- **40 g of corn malt**
- **40 ml of corn oil**
- **5 g of fresh brewer's yeast**
- **the grated rind of 1 lemon**
- **60 ml of warm water**

Berries cream:
- **250 g of corn malt**
- **200 g of berries**
- **50 g of corn starch**
- **250 ml of cold water**
- **1 pinch of salt**

Start by preparing the berry cream: put the malt, the washed berries, 200 ml of water, and a pinch of salt in a pot. Cook over low heat and mix. Meanwhile, in a bowl, dissolve the corn starch with the remaining water. When the berries reach boiling point, add the water with the dissolved starch and mix with a whisk to prevent lumps from forming. Within a few minutes, the cream thickens: turn off the heat and pour it into a large baking dish to let it cool. Then proceed with the preparation of the dough for the cake. Put all the dry ingredients in a bowl: flour, salt, and lemon peel and mix them. Then form a hole in the center and mix in the corn oil, kneading it with a bit of dough. Also, add the malt and yeast: work carefully, helping yourself with a bit of flour until you get a homogeneous ball.

Continue to knead for a few minutes on a floured work surface: the result must be a smooth and elastic mixture that you will leave to rest covered with a cloth for 30 minutes.

With a rolling pin, roll out the pastry forming a 30 cm disk, place it on a baking sheet lined with baking paper and shape the edge. Pour in the cold berry cream. Bake in a preheated oven at 200 ° for 40 minutes, until the surface is golden brown.

•Cocoa pudding

Ingredients:
- **500 ml of soy milk**
- **4 tablespoons of unsweetened cocoa**
- **3-4 tablespoons of brown sugar**
- **2 tablespoons of corn starch**
- **1 pinch of natural vanilla**
- **chopped hazelnuts to decorate**

Sift the cocoa, starch, and sugar; collect them in a saucepan together with vanilla. First, add 100 ml of milk, stirring well to remove all lumps, and then the rest. Over medium heat, bring to a boil without stopping stirring. Lower the heat and cook for a couple of minutes more until the mixture has thickened. Moisten four single-portion molds and pour the pudding. Let it cool down and put it in the fridge until completely cooled. Decorate with the grains and serve.

•Bavarian yogurt with pumpkin

Ingredients:
- **350 ml of natural yogurt**
- **150 g of grated pumpkin**
- **1 tablespoon of honey**
- **1 tablespoon of agar-agar**
- **1 pinch of salt**

Pour the pumpkin into a saucepan with 100 ml of yogurt, salt, and agar-agar; cook for 5 minutes. Remove from heat, let cool and add the remaining yogurt, honey. Stir the mixture well, then pour it into the bowls and let it cool to room temperature or in the refrigerator.

•Quinoa pralines with peach pulp

Ingredients:
- **1 ripe yellow peach**
- **150 g of quinoa**
- **2 tablespoons of brown sugar**
- **7 tablespoons of coconut flour**
- **5 tablespoons of chopped peanuts**

Peel the peach and chop the pulp in the mixer until you get a homogeneous cream that you will put in the fridge. Rinse the quinoa well under running water and cook it in a pot with boiling water for the package's time. When cooked, drain it, put it in a bowl, add the sugar and let it cool completely. Add with the coconut flour and the peach cream until you get a thick and compact mixture that you will work with your hands to make balls with a diameter of about 3-4 centimeters. Roll them in chopped peanuts and put them in the freezer for 20 minutes, then transfer them to the fridge and always serve them cold.

•Strawberry Tofu Mousse

Ingredients:
- **200 g of natural tofu**
- **250 g of strawberries**
- **3 tablespoons of 100% gluten-free rice or corn malt**
- **chocolate flakes**
- **some mint leaves**
- **1 tablespoon of lemon juice**
- **water as required**

Prepare a mint infusion by leaving the leaves to infuse for at least ten minutes in hot water. Strain it and use that water to boil the tofu together with three tablespoons of malt for a few minutes. After cooking, let the mixture cool in its water to make it flavor well. Drain and blend the tofu with the clean and chopped strawberries and a tablespoon of lemon juice. Use the infusion water to help you combine the tofu and strawberries well and obtain a soft mousse. Pour the cream into the cups and store it in the refrigerator for an hour. Finally, garnish with fresh mint leaves and chocolate flakes.

• Chocolate pears

Ingredients:
- **1 kg of pears**
- **a little cinnamon or vanilla**
- **100 g of bitter chocolate**
- **3 tablespoons of honey**

Peel the pears, halve them and remove the core. Put them in a saucepan with cinnamon or vanilla and cook them slightly covered with water. Then transfer them to a serving dish, keeping the cooking water. Melt 3 tablespoons of honey in a saucepan and pour it over the pears. In its place, put the chopped chocolate with a little cooking water from the pears. Let it melt until smooth, adding more cooking water if necessary. Spread it over the pears and serve.

•Coconut balls

Ingredients:
- **1 cup of peanuts**
- **5 dates**
- **grated coconut to taste**
- **rice milk to taste**

Pitted the dates, cut them into small pieces, put them in a robot together with the peanuts, and blended them finely. With your hands, form balls, compacting them well. Let them rest for half an hour in the fridge. Meanwhile, mix a little coconut with two tablespoons of rice milk. Take the balls back and roll them in this mixture until they are evenly covered. Finally, put them in the paper cups and serve them.

Creams, sauces, dressings

•Broccoli cream

Ingredients:
- **300 g of broccoli stalks**
- **2 shallots**
- **½ teaspoon of marjoram**
- **30 g of shelled walnuts**
- **vegetable broth**
- **4 tablespoons of oil**
- **salt and chilli**

Peel the stems with a potato peeler and steam them until tender (about 20 minutes). Meanwhile, finely chop the shallots and put them in a pan with half the oil and the same water amount. Add the chili pepper according to taste, marjoram, and a pinch of salt. Let them soften over low heat, stirring occasionally; finally, raise the heat and let the liquid evaporate. When the broccoli stems are warm, pass them to the mixer with the rest of the oil and enough broth to have a homogeneous cream and a little fluid. Add the ground walnuts and the shallots, season with salt and serve the hot cream to season a pasta plate.

•Strawberry jam

Ingredients:
• 1 kg of well-ripened and healthy organic strawberries
• the juice of 1 lemon
• 100 grams of whole cane sugar
• 1 teaspoon of vanilla powder

Wash and cut the strawberries into wedges, sprinkle with lemon juice, add vanilla and sprinkle with sugar. Let them macerate in this aromatic mixture for an hour. After this time, put them in a saucepan, and simmer for 30-40 minutes, stirring often, and let them rest for 15 minutes. Boil the mixture for a few more minutes and put it still hot in new and sterilized jars. Then heat the jars in a pot for 30 minutes, then let them cool upside down side by side and covered with a tea towel. Check when they have cooled down if the cap is closed correctly. Place in a place away from heat or sunlight and in a cool place.

• Tofu cream with zucchini and mint

Ingredients:
- **100 g of tofu**
- **1 spring onion**
- **2 small or 1 large zucchini**
- **1 handful of mint leaves**
- **1 pinch of whole salt**
- **1 tablespoon of extra virgin olive oil**
- **2 tablespoons of water**
- **½ tablespoon of soy mayonnaise**

Prepare the vegetables for cooking: wash the zucchini and trim them, peel the spring onion. Grate the first with the special tool with large holes and finely chop the second. Sauté them both in a pan for 6 minutes with the oil and water. Meanwhile, chop the aromatic herbs and mix them with the contents of the pan. Also, add the crumbled tofu, salt, and continue cooking for another 5 minutes. Allow to cool and serve on bread with soy mayonnaise.

•Beetroot sauce

Ingredients:
- **1 small raw beetroot**
- **1 small shallot**
- **100 g of smoked or plain tofu**
- **4 juniper berries**
- **2 tablespoons of sunflower seeds**
- **salt a pinch**

Simmer the tofu in lightly salted water for a few minutes. Drain it and place it in the blender. Peel and clean the beetroot and cut it into small chunks. Clean the shallot. Pour the beetroot and chopped shallot into the blender with the tofu, then add the juniper berries, sunflower seeds, and salt. Blend everything. If necessary, blend the sauce, help yourself with a bit of tofu cooking water or a drizzle of extra virgin olive oil. The sauce can be served with hot croutons or as a sauce for pasta. Alternatively, it is excellent for filling pancakes.

•Custard cream

Ingredients:
•600 g of soy milk
•80 g of raw cane sugar
•30 grams of flour 0
•18 g of corn starch
•1 gram of powdered agar-agar
•1 tablespoon of sunflower oil
•the zest of 1 organic lemon
•half a sachet of saffron

Put the sifted flour and corn starch in a bowl, add the saffron and the agar-agar, jumbled up. Pour in 100 g of soy milk, constantly stirring well with a whisk to not form lumps, and leave aside. Gather the rest of the milk and sugar in a saucepan. Flavor with lemon zest (only the yellow outer part) and simmer over medium heat. Lower the heat and pour in the flour and starch mixture, constantly stirring with a whisk for about 3 minutes. Add the oil, mix, and immediately transfer the cream into a bowl and cover with baking paper. Cool the cream and work it briefly with a spatula or spoon before using it.

Note: fundamental base for fillings, desserts by the glass, tiramisu.

•Guacamole

Ingredients:
- •Ripe avocado 1
- •Green chilli 1
- •Copper tomatoes 1
- •Extra virgin olive oil 20 g
- •Lime juice 10 g
- •Shallot 10 g
- •Black pepper 1 pinch
- •Salt up to 1 pinch

Start by looking after the avocado. Cut it in half lengthwise, then sink the knife's blade into the core and pull to extract it easily. Cut the pulp with a small knife to remove it more easily with a spoon; collect it in a small bowl. Then cut the lime in half and squeeze it to obtain the juice, be poured on the avocado pulp; Then, season with salt and pepper, and mash the pulp with a fork. Set aside, then peel and finely chop the shallot, then wash, dry, and slice the tomato: obtained from the cubes' slices. Then tick the green (or red) chili pepper, empty it of its seeds, cut it into strips, and then into cubes. Then in the bowl with the crushed avocado pulp, pour the chopped shallot and the diced tomatoes. Also, add the chili and oil, stir and add more salt and pepper if necessary. Your guacamole sauce is ready to be enjoyed!

•Fresh tomato sauce with basil

Ingredients:
•Copper tomatoes 1.2 kg
•Extra virgin olive oil 3 tbsp
•Salt up to taste
•Basil 8 leaves

Remove the stalks and wash them very well, then dry them. Cut each tomato into two halves and remove the green part of each of them' stem. Squeeze the two halves of the tomato into a bowl or sink so that all the seeds come out. Put the tomatoes in a steel pot, which you will arrange on low heat covered by the lid; let the tomatoes cook, turning them from time to time until they are wilted and come apart. Pass the tomatoes with a vegetable mill making the sauce converge in a bowl; once all the tomatoes have been passed, pour the sauce into a smaller steel pot that you will put on the stove. Add the salt and oil to the sauce, consume it over high heat to the desired density, turn off the heat, and add the whole basil or coarsely chopped by hand. Perfect with spaghetti!

•Herbal sauce

Ingredients:
- **1 bunch of aromatic herbs**
- **2 tablespoons of extra virgin olive oil**
- **200 ml of fresh cream vegetable**
- **salt**
- **pepper**

First, wash the chosen herbs (I used basil, rosemary, parsley, and mint), dry them, remove the stems, and chop them. Once chopped, put them in a bowl and add salt, pepper, cream, and oil, then emulsify well with a fork. The herb sauce is ready; you can use it immediately or keep it in the fridge.

•Chestnut cream

Ingredients:
•Chestnuts 2 kg
•Brown Sugar Br 600 g
•Water 650 ml
•Untreated lemon zest 1
•Vanilla bean 1

Start by washing the chestnuts under running water, then place them whole in a pot full of water and boil them for at least 15 minutes, then drain and let them cool. At this point, peel the chestnuts with a sharp knife. Transfer the chestnuts to the vegetable mill to obtain a sandy mixture, or you can use the potato masher. In this way, you will get about 1.6 kg of pulp. Now take the vanilla pod, cut it lengthwise, and extract the internal seeds. Place a pan with a high edge on the stove, add the vanilla pod with its seeds, sugar, and water. Melt the sugar over medium heat, stirring with a whisk for about 10 minutes. When the sugar is completely dissolved, remove the vanilla pod with kitchen tongs and stir in the chestnuts and mix the mixture. Grate the zest of an untreated lemon and add it to the cream. Cook over low heat for about 1 hour, occasionally stirring with a wooden spoon. The chestnut cream will be ready when it becomes a creamy puree. At this point, pour the chestnut cream into the jars with a spoon; your chestnut cream is prepared.

•Coconut milk cream

Ingredients:
•Coconut milk 400 ml
•Sugar 50 g
•Rice flour 20 g

Start by pouring the sugar and rice flour into a saucepan. Then add the coconut milk a little at a time, continually stirring with a whisk. Place on the heat and continue stirring until you reach the desired density, then move from the heat and continue stirring. Pour the mixture into a bowl. Cover with the cling film and let cool before enjoying your coconut cream.

Conclusion

About 50 million US citizens have thyroid problems. The thyroid is a butterfly-shaped gland found in the front of our neck, between the larynx and the trachea. Although small in size, the thyroid has a fundamental role in our body because the hormones it produces, called thyroid hormones, are necessary for numerous growth and development functions, such as regulating metabolism, body temperature, and muscle strength. Its alteration has negative and significant consequences on the quality of life. The causes of thyroid alteration can be numerous but the most frequent, in addition to the genetic ones, are hyperthyroidism and hypothyroidism, allergies, metabolic diseases, prolonged radiation exposure. To protect this precious gland's health, it is essential to follow, in addition to the appropriate medical and pharmacological indications, a healthy and balanced diet.